COPING WITH SUICIDE

Signs We Missed and Strategies To Use In The Aftermath

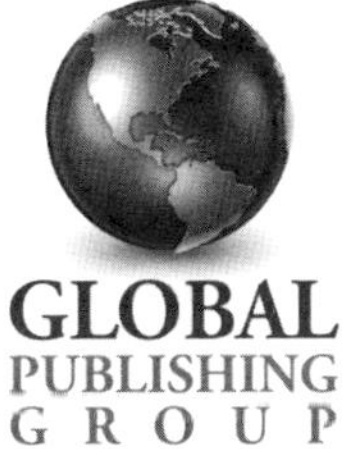

Global Publishing Group
Australia • New Zealand • Singapore • America • London

COPING WITH SUICIDE

Signs We Missed and Strategies To Use In The Aftermath

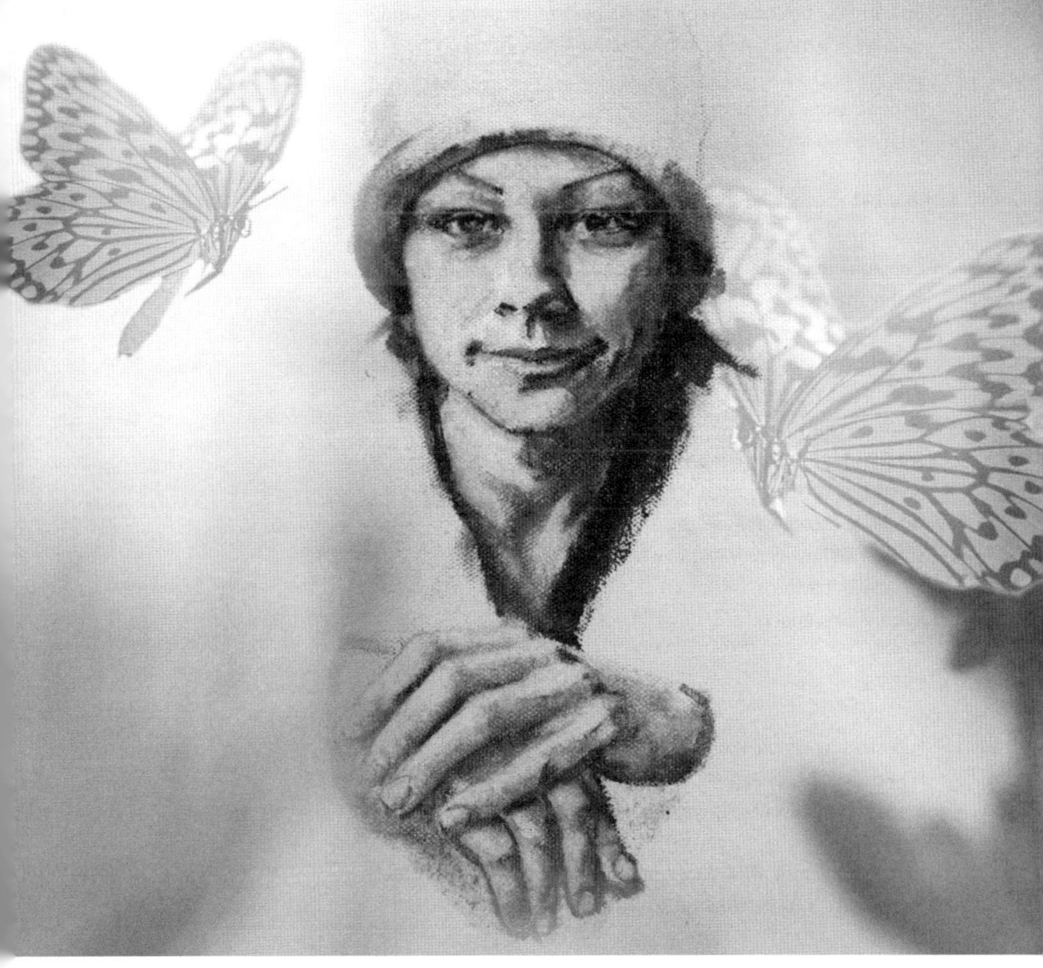

CHRISTINE J HOWARD

DISCLAIMER

All the information, techniques, skills and concepts contained within this publication are of the nature of general comment only and are not in any way recommended as individual advice. The intent is to offer a variety of information to provide a wider range of choices now and in the future, recognising that we all have widely diverse circumstances and viewpoints. Should any reader choose to make use of the information contained herein, this is their decision, and the contributors (and their companies), authors and publishers do not assume any responsibilities whatsoever under any condition or circumstances. It is recommended that the reader obtain their own independent advice.

First Edition 2015

Copyright © 2015 Christine J Howard

All rights are reserved. The material contained within this book is protected by copyright law, no part may be copied, reproduced, presented, stored, communicated or transmitted in any form by any means without prior written permission..

National Library of Australia
Cataloguing-in-Publication entry:

Howard, Christine J., 1952- author.

Coping with suicide : signs we missed and strategies to use
in the aftermath / Christine J Howard.

1st ed.
ISBN: 9781922118844 (paperback)

Suicide--Psychological aspects.
Bereavement--Psychological aspects.
Grief--Psychological aspects.
Suicide victims--Family relationships.
Suicidal behavior.
Suicide--Prevention.

362.283

Published by Global Publishing Group
PO Box 517 Mt Evelyn, Victoria 3796 Australia
Email info@GlobalPublishingGroup.com.au

For further information about orders:
Phone: +61 3 9739 4686 or Fax +61 3 8648 6871

This book is dedicated to my family, particularly my husband Ross: thank you for hanging in there with me through all the ups and downs of the past 40-plus years, for supporting and bolstering me when I doubted myself.

Also to my awesome children Matthew and Fiona, and their wonderful spouses, Quill and Damian, who encouraged me to write this story.

Also to my grandchildren – Joshua, Hayley, Ezekiel and Gabriel – just for being you.

Thank you all for believing in me. Without that, this book would not have been possible.

And of course to my beautiful, fun-loving Kelly, who was the inspiration for this book.

Christine J Howard

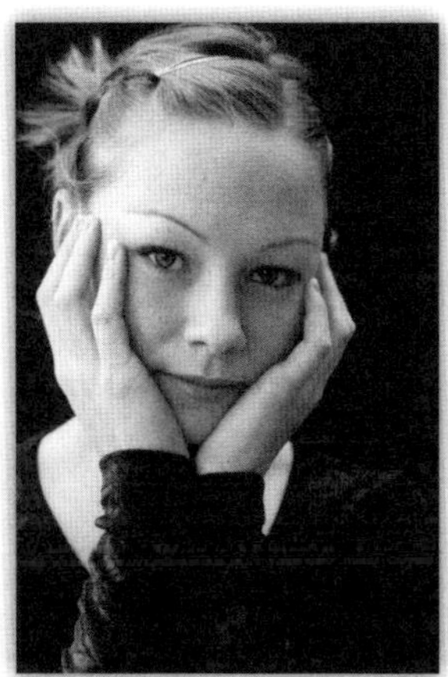

ACKNOWLEDGEMENTS

Firstly I'd like to acknowledge my son Matthew for painting the beautiful portrait of Kelly (on the cover).

I would like to thank my father-in-law Peter for his very generous support in getting this book published.

I also wish to thank the Wednesday girls for their support and encouragement and for keeping me grounded. Julie, Sharon and Marion – I love you heaps!

Also thanks to Susan and Pauline – the best neighbours to have in a crisis.

Thanks to Jen for the amazing help in editing, making my words into a real book.

I'd also like to acknowledge the care and compassion shown by the police and ambulance personnel, in particular Ted H from the Geelong Police Station.

Thank you too to those of you who shared insights into how it feels when you decide suicide is the way to go, and who thankfully didn't take that path.

And to those who offered encouragement, and who supported us through the really dark times – too many of you to name – you helped us all to survive the worst times.

Last, but not least, to Ross who really helped make all this possible.

CONTENTS

CHAPTER 1

Why This Book? My Reflections

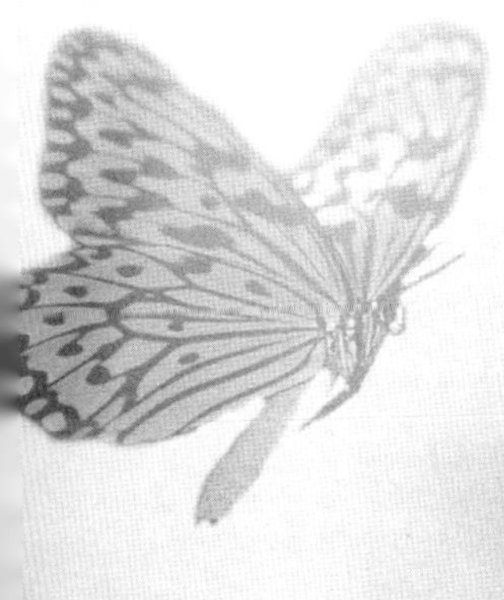

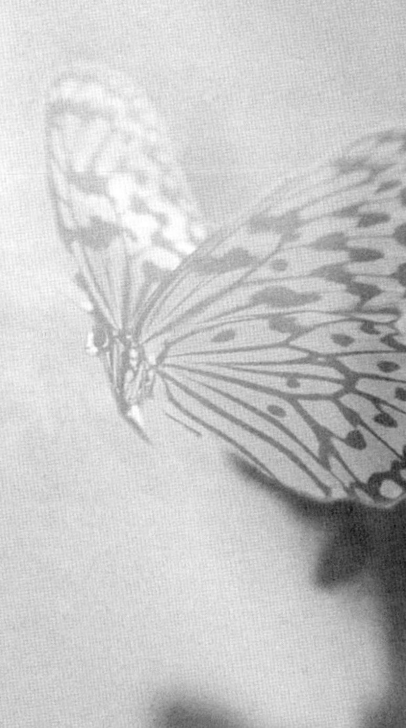

MASKS

You probably won't recognise me today
Because I have taken off my many masks.

You have never met me before and
Nor have you ever seen me this way.

So hello my dear friend, at last we finally meet,
I have uncovered myself to introduce you to me.

Feel free to walk away and leave me in this crazy world.
For I may have the urge to do so myself.

And if by chance I do leave you,
I want you to know that it is forever ... Goodbye.

Kelly Howard, 11 September 1995

CHAPTER 1
Why This Book? My Reflections

Some days it's just really hard to function normally.

I go through the motions of living, answer the phone, hold conversations, and probably appear to be doing OK. But inside I just feel empty. I think about how nice it would be to just get away from everyone and not have to talk. Somewhere I could simply read a novel and escape from the world for a while. Or maybe just go out and get some sunshine, to take a walk along the beach.

The rational, logical part of my mind tells me to stop it, to get on with life and stop feeling sorry for myself.

Then there's the melancholy part, the sad part that means I simply exist in a state of sadness. And really, it's OK to feel this way.

Grief has no time limit, and I guess some days are meant to be reflective. A time where I can just be sad, without making a major issue out of it all.

Unfortunately some of those days can get me thinking in a really negative, almost self-destructive way.

Doubts creep in and it can be difficult believing in myself in any way except a negative one. Questions run through my mind in a repetitive loop:

- Why would anyone want to read a book I've written?
- What sort of a mother am I that I wasn't able to help my daughter?

- How can I possibly think that I could help other families from going through what we went through?
- Who'd want to listen to me?
- I'm not a very nice person, am I?
- Who do I think I am?

Sometimes I even wonder if all this is worth it.

But then sanity prevails, bringing me back to reality and I start counting my blessings again. Somehow, amazingly, the doubts begin to fade. Reality steps in and I realise that I'm just wallowing again, and that's OK. Then I take a deep breath and just "be" in the moment with who I am.

I know that I'm not a failure. I know that I have faced some rather big obstacles in my life, and I have survived despite them. I know that I will keep on surviving, because I believe I have a message to share.

Fairly early on after Kelly's death, Ross and I came up with the simple phrase "I'm just having an attack of the Kellys," to account for our feelings. It saved us trying to explain that we weren't feeling in top shape, but it also meant that we understood each other, and we allowed one another the time to just be with those feelings.

We, each and every one, deal with our grief in different ways, possibly simply because we are females or males. There is no right way to grieve; what works for one may not work for another.

Early on for me it was often a glass of wine with friends or family – I stopped short of drinking alone, scared that it may become a crutch to lean on.

I recall often coming home from work, getting out of my car and hearing the stereo blaring with a song that Ross associated with Kelly. I'd come in to find him sitting with numerous small tea light candles lit around the decking, beer in hand, listening to the music.

In the beginning, I would mentally roll my eyes, take a deep breath and brace myself to deal with "that" Ross. And then I realised my selfishness for judging how Ross was dealing with his grief. Just because he didn't handle it the way I did didn't mean he was wrong. It was just his way. Once I came to that conclusion and stopped being the judge and jury, it was easy.

For me it was often easier to write down my feelings, so I would get out my journal and pour them out onto the page. I wrote many letters to Kelly, sharing day-to-day happenings, as I had when she was alive. It was a strategy or coping mechanism, as I immersed myself in my writing to minimise the pain I was going through. I have included some of these letters to show my feelings at the time, and how we were coping.

Sometime in the early weeks after Kelly died, I voiced my growing thought that she had died for a reason, but I just didn't know what that reason was at the time.

As a parent grieving for a beloved daughter, I went through all the usual mental discussions. I rationalised the why, clutching at any explanation that could give hope. Surely it wasn't all for nothing. Her life was worth so much more than to be just a brief memory to her friends and teachers, and a more lasting one to her family.

Now I believe that the reason for her death was for me to write this book.

For years my children have teased me about my book – the one that I've been saying I would write someday. I didn't know what I would write about, but I knew that I would do it some day. So then I began to think about writing Kelly's story. Then I wondered if anyone would really want to read another sad story.

So many people have lost loved ones to suicide; why should our story be any different?

But the belief has been growing inside, getting gradually stronger in me for the last fourteen or so years.

Well, this is the time. My someday. When I knew I was ready, the opportunity appeared. By the time it came, I believed that by telling Kelly's story, I could possibly help other families who have suffered a loss like ours, maybe even save a life. Although I may not necessarily know whether this happens, it doesn't really matter.

I began to think about the perception of suicide, and how it is still shrouded in such mystique.

There are still questions surrounding suicide. Although it is now discussed much more openly, and there is a substantial amount of help available, there are still far too many lives lost to this devastating act.

We've come a long way from the days where it wasn't talked about at all, when, if someone had taken their own life, they were buried in "unconsecrated ground", out of the churchyard cemetery where people were normally buried. Where the stigma of suicide was synonymous with shame.

People went to great lengths to disguise the fact that a loved one had taken their own life, and some of that secrecy has lingered on today.

So we talk a lot more about suicide, and that is making a difference I'm sure, but there are still far too many deaths for us to be comfortable with it.

Too many misconceptions around the "whys"; and then too much guilt for loved ones who regret not taking the "right" action. I guess that will always be there, as many who die by suicide are masters of disguise. They hide their distress from loved ones, possibly hoping to spare them pain, but ending up causing so much more suffering with the never-to-be-answered questions.

My intention in sharing Kelly's story is to raise awareness around suicide. To dispel some of the myths associated with this scourge on our society. It's a big ask I know, but if I can help just one family to recognise that there are steps that anyone can take that may help prevent another tragedy, then this book has been worthwhile.

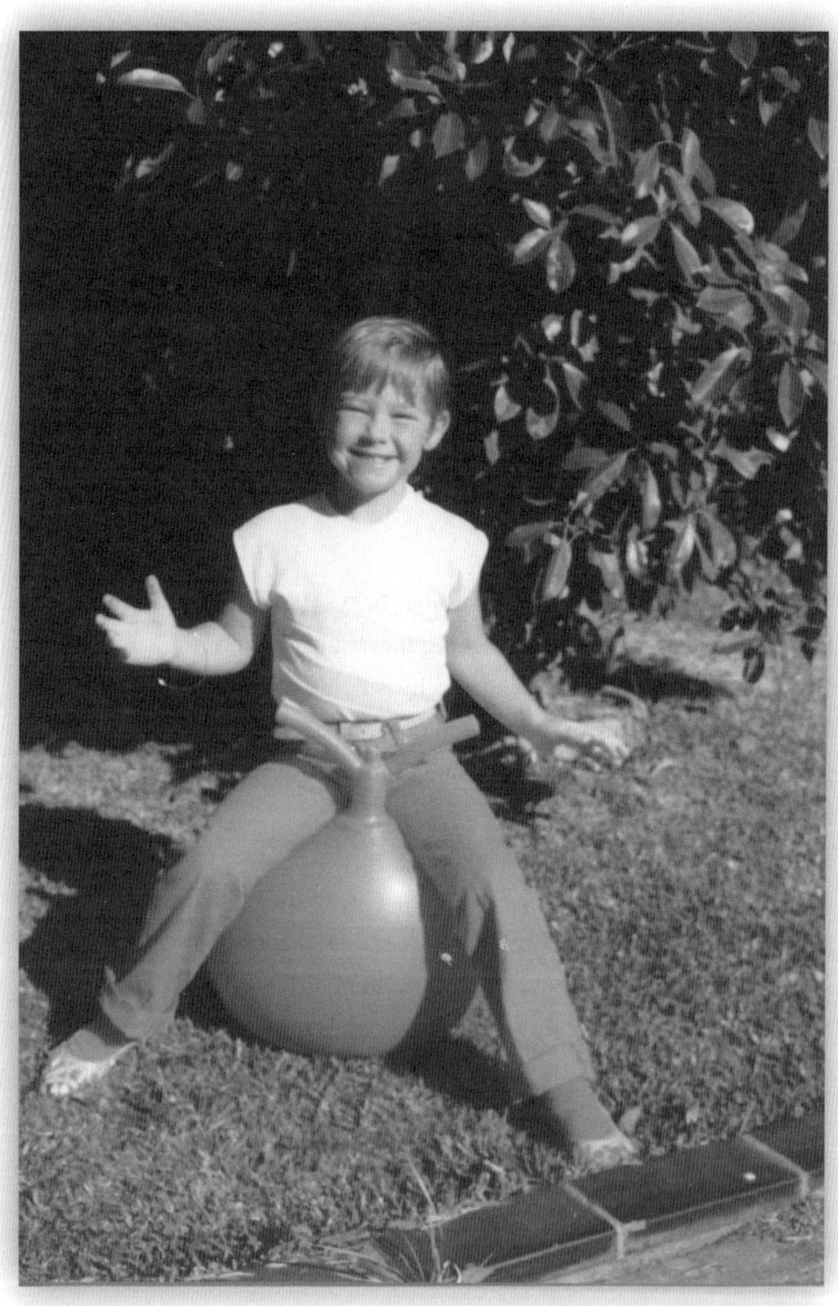

CHAPTER 2

About Kelly

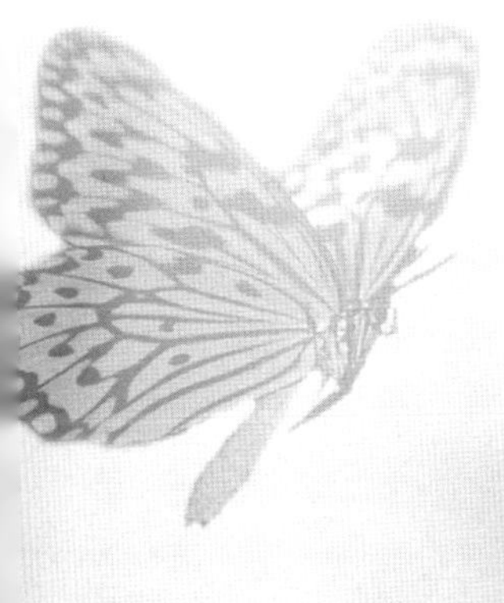

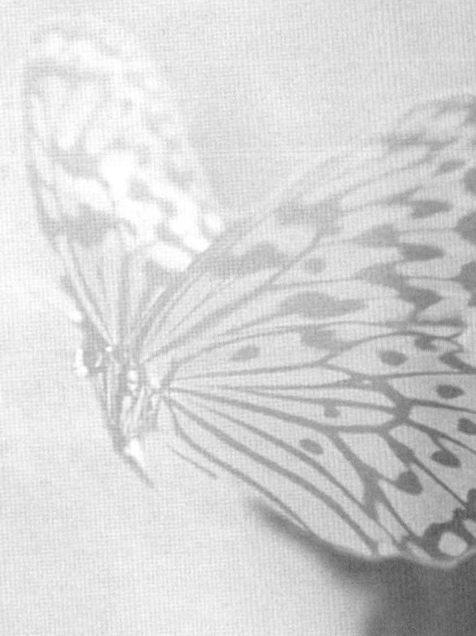

KELLY

Keep a goal in mind,
When life's not very kind.
Just hold on to your dream,
And though at times you'll seem
To just be standing still,
When nothing seems to thrill.
Just keep on keeping on,
Maybe then you will have won.

Christine Howard 11 November 1997

CHAPTER 2
About Kelly

I spent a good part of the early hours of Remembrance Day 1979 in a labour ward at Box Hill Hospital. Ross was by my side, wiping my sweaty brow and attempting to soothe me (and shushing me as I swore) when I just wanted it all over and done with.

I'd done this twice before and had a fair idea of the routine, but when the obstetrician finally arrived (apologising as he'd forgotten the early-morning call telling him I was there), he decided on a forceps delivery. As the baby was pulled into the world all I could see was the head of black hair. And then the announcement, "It's a girl!"

If I hadn't seen her being born, I would never have believed she was one of mine, as the other two had almost invisible blond fluff on their heads when they were born.

The name "Kelly" was one Ross and I had chosen for a girl, but we couldn't decide on a second one. Ross's Mum suggested "Christine", so she was named Kelly Christine.

Someone enquired later if I'd observed the minute's silence for Remembrance Day, to which I replied, "No, I think I was swearing at that time."

Life was rather busy, as Kelly was born one week before Matthew turned three and Fiona was almost 15 months old. Still, it was simply my life at the time and, although it was hectic, there was no point in complaining.

Kelly endured being carted around in her carry basket, propped in the middle of the backseat of the station wagon in between the two car seats. (Our generation showed an amazing disregard for safety in this area!)

One of the toys gifted to Kelly when she was born was a pink teddy bear. It became her favorite and she was seldom without it. Tipping Pink Teddy upside down, holding one leg in her hand Kelly would gently rub the foot back and forth under her nose whilst sucking her thumb.

Pink Teddy was her comforter, best friend and sleep mate. Pink Teddy became so worn and threadbare, that when he couldn't be mended anymore, I had to make him a tracksuit to keep the stuffing inside.

Kelly's childhood was quite ordinary; we moved from Melbourne back to Geelong when she was three. She attended kindergarten in Geelong West, and then Ashby Primary School where she was a diligent student.

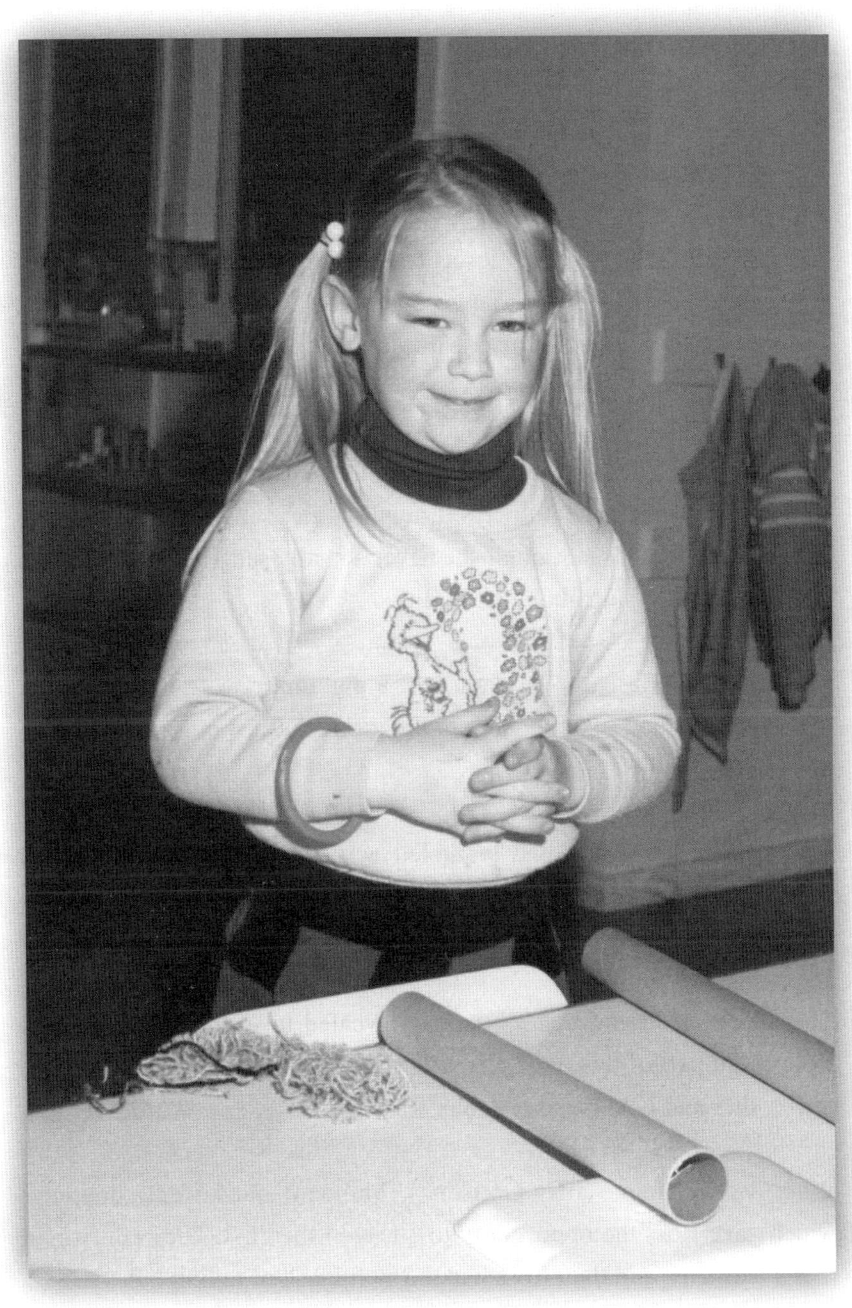

High school was Matthew Flinders Secondary College. Going to parent–teacher interviews was almost a waste of time as, with the exception of one teacher in high school, Kelly received the glowing reports of an A-grade student. Kell was a bit of a perfectionist.

Kelly did all the usual activities as a child: calisthenics, Brownies, Girl Guides and netball. She was an excellent netballer and received several awards over the years. She also learnt to play the flute in high school.

Poetry was a favored pastime, and Kelly used this means of expression over the years. She had aspirations of being an actor, and participated in many drama activities and plays throughout her school years. She also took singing lessons, although she never actually sang for the family, so we were left guessing about her ability.

Christmas 1989 was the beginning of a nightmare, with the revelation that my father had sexually abused the girls. Not just our girls, but also most in my family.

My sister-in-law Anne had stumbled across a letter from my niece written to *Dolly* magazine. It told the story of her abuse at Dad's hands, and opened up the whole can of worms.

The family gathering that Christmas revealed to Anne that Fiona and Kelly were part of this dark secret. Unsure of how to break the news to my brother and I, Anne confided in Ross.

When we got home after Christmas, Matthew and I went shopping, which gave Ross the opportunity to question the girls. They confirmed that it was true, and then Ross had the awful task of telling me.

The girls were in bed and Ross sat me down to tell me. At first I didn't believe it. How could the man I respected and loved have destroyed my children's innocence? Then I rationalised it by saying that perhaps the girls had misunderstood, making much more of it than needed to be.

Ross and I went into the bedroom to see the girls, and he asked them to tell me. I'm ashamed to say now that I wasn't a very supportive mother initially.

Kelly asked, "If it happened to us, did it happen to you?" I said no, and she asked "Why not?" I said I didn't know, but I had no memories of anything like that.

That night I couldn't stop thinking about it, and began to remember bits and pieces of conversations with my mother. She'd told of their church minister speaking to Dad about his behaviour with some of the girls at youth group, which Dad ran at the church. The pieces were adding up, and I felt so betrayed when the awful reality of it all finally sank in. As it happened that minister was now living in Geelong, so the next day I called him and told him what I knew, still hoping that it was all a horrible nightmare. His response was, "Christine, I'm not surprised."

I asked him what to do. I was not equipped to handle anything like this, and I knew I needed to get professional help for us all, especially the girls. This was to be the start of a roller-coaster of emotions for all of us, with visits to counsellors and feelings of utter devastation that my beautiful children had been violated. Child abuse was something that happened in other families, and it was so hard to accept that it had happened in mine.

At the time, it seemed that the girls were coping reasonably well with it all. They went to counselling for a while, then informed me that they were alright now and didn't need to go anymore. I couldn't force them to keep going, so just had to hope that Ross and I would be able to help them enough.

The early teen years seemed to be particularly difficult, although I didn't really have a "normal" yardstick to measure that with. Perhaps it just seemed that way. I strongly believe that the abuse had a big influence on the girls' teen years.

Fiona and Kelly were very close, not just in age – there was only fifteen months between them – but I think more because of their shared experiences at Dad's hands.

In 1994 after another teenage argument, Fiona left home. It was an extremely stressful time for all of us, but particularly hard for Kelly, as she and Fiona were so close.

Kelly and I kept tabs on where Fiona was and whom she was staying with, and we were able to meet with her regularly. During the day at school Kelly would follow up leads and then come home and we would make phone calls checking to see if she was all right or if she needed anything.

Then Fiona moved in with her best friend "J", and her family. Not long afterwards she contracted a really bad cold, so I went to the pharmacy and bought cough medicine and a large bottle of paracetamol for her. She may not have been at home, but at least I could still look after her in some way.

Then there was an issue with her girlfriend and her parents, who took J out of school and sent her to Ballarat. Fiona rang me then and said she wanted to come home, and asked if I could pick her up.

I picked her up and stuffed all of her clothes and bedding into the back of my mini. We were on our way home when she suddenly decided that she needed to catch up with some friends in town. So I reluctantly dropped her off and went home to wait for her call to be picked up again.

She rang later to say that she was going to stay with friends in Leopold, and that she would be home the next day. I wasn't too happy about that, but there wasn't much I could do but accept it.

Just after midnight that night, we received a phone call from the hospital to say that Fiona had been admitted following an overdose. She'd apparently taken most of the tablets I'd bought. Later we heard that the hospital only called because the friend who had found her had insisted that her parents should know she was there.

It was such a shock, totally unexpected and very hard on Kelly.

Fiona stayed overnight in hospital; Ross and I accompanied Fiona to the ward. She had an intravenous drip up, and seemed reasonably OK. I returned in the morning to visit, having made a quick stop at my work to see my boss and ask which psychiatrist I should request if needed. I had a feeling that the hospital would be insisting on psychiatric intervention.

When I arrived, Fiona was sitting up in bed. She asked me to help her go for a shower. She got out of bed and I wheeled the IV pole and its attached IMED pump across to the bathroom. As I disconnected the pump to make it easier for her to move, a nurse came into the room, looked at us, but made no comment on the fact that the IMED had been disconnected, then just turned and left.

I was feeling rather angry that no one had bothered to take Fiona's jeans off and put her in a gown. She even had an imprint on her hip of the cigarette lighter that was still in her pocket.

I felt disgusted and ashamed that my nursing colleagues could treat a young girl this way. They had passed judgment on her because she'd attempted suicide. Nobody deigned to ask why or what had brought her to that point. They just treated her as a nuisance, a time waster.

That morning Fiona was visited by several officious men in white coats – interns I suppose – who told Ross and me to step outside the room as they were pulling the curtains around Fiona's bed. Ross and I did as we were told, and waited in the corridor. Then one white-coated man came up and started telling us how serious this situation was. I stopped him and asked who he was, and did he realise that my daughter was a private patient? He was surprised, and apologised saying that he hadn't realised.

Later that day Fiona saw the psychiatrist, and then I was able to see him as well. He told me that while she had refused to say she wouldn't attempt suicide again, there was nothing more he could do so he was discharging her. I was stunned, and said, "You mean to tell me that you're going to let my daughter go when she has said she might do this again?" I cried then, and said, " She refuses to come home to live, so I may never see her again!" The psychiatrist replied that the only way he could keep her was perhaps to transfer her to the psychiatric ward, but he wasn't sure he could.

I went home that evening, not knowing if Fiona would be discharged or transferred to the psych ward, and wondering whether she would be successful with the next suicide attempt.

Another stressor to add into the mix was having my mother also in the hospital as an inpatient. I was juggling visiting her and Fiona, but at least the charge nurse on Mum's ward was very helpful and caring, perhaps because we'd worked together a few years before.

When I rang the ward the next morning I was informed that Fiona wasn't there anymore. My heart sank as I thought they'd let her go, but then they said she'd been transferred to Dax House – the psychiatric ward. After two days there, Fiona called me and asked me to take her home again – to live in the caravan – a compromise.

Early on in our counselling sessions with Margaret, Margaret explained to me that there are generally two types of responses to sexual abuse. Some girls become very introverted, and often put on weight, whilst others may become rather promiscuous. I seemed to have one of each.

In 1995 Fiona gave birth to Joshua, and Kelly fell in love with him. She was his devoted aunt, and absolutely adored him.

In 1996, Year 11, Kelly made her debut. I had made her deb dress, which she was so proud of. It was a lovely night, followed by the afterparty at our house. The decking was groaning with a seething mass of teenagers, and it was so much fun.

It was an eventful year, and halfway through Kelly succumbed to a particularly virulent chest infection. She was quite ill, and at one stage was coughing so hard she had burst blood vessels in both eyes. Eventually she was diagnosed with chronic fatigue, and missed the better part of terms three and four.

With her record of being such a good student, the school decided that she didn't need to repeat year 11, but could progress to year 12. However, year 12 was very demanding, and having missed so much school the year before, Kelly was unable to keep up. This was very demoralising for her as she struggled to do the work to her exacting standards.

Back at school, Kelly seemed to be coping quite well, until she called me at work after school one day. She was weepy saying, "Mum, I've taken too many pills!" My heart began pounding with fear, I said I was coming, dropped what I was doing, hastily told my colleague that I was going home as Kelly was unwell, and raced to my car.

It was a slow trip home – at least it seemed that way, as I had to negotiate the after-school traffic. I wasn't sure what I would find when I got home and started berating myself for not calling an ambulance right away.

When I got home, I found Kelly lying on the sofa, very apologetic. She said she'd vomited and was feeling better. She'd even cleaned up after herself, and her towels were soaking in the laundry sink.

I wasn't convinced so rang our doctor and asked what I should do. She told me to get an ambulance anyway as Kelly needed to be assessed. The ambulance came and took her to hospital, where she was admitted for the night.

It was rather hectic, as Ross and I were looking after Joshua at the time. I'd dropped him off at his daycare on my way to work that morning, and was meant to collect him after work. I called them and they were happy to keep him until they closed later that evening, so we were able to concentrate on Kelly for a few hours.

For some reason, we didn't have to go down the path of psychiatric consultations like we had with Fiona, perhaps because it wasn't considered as serious as Fiona's attempt. We brought Kelly home the next day, and she seemed to recover OK. There were counseling sessions, but I'm not sure how much good they did.

During one conversation I had with Kelly, she told me that there wasn't one day that she didn't think of the abuse. This was around the time she was writing lots of poetry; I suppose it was a way of coping with the burden of what her grandfather had done to her.

STRONGER

I totally lack self-confidence.
I'm not sure why.
Perhaps my childhood didn't help.
I wish I was emotionally stronger,
But I'm not.
I feel like breaking down and crying every day of my life.
It's just over the little things that I don't feel comfortable with.
How can I grow stronger?
I know I need to.
But how?

Kelly Howard, 1996

CHAPTER 3

The Beginning of the End

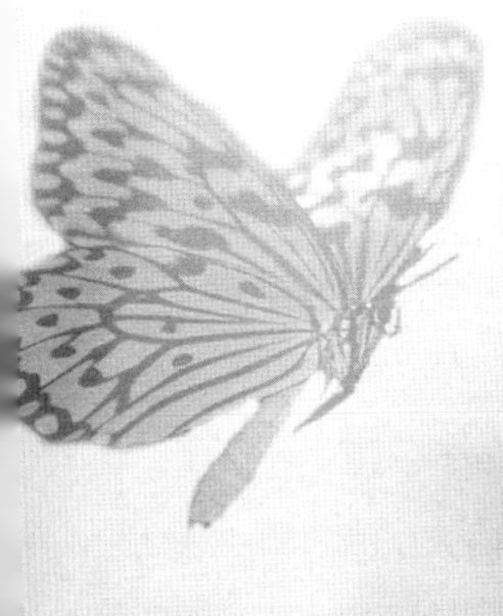

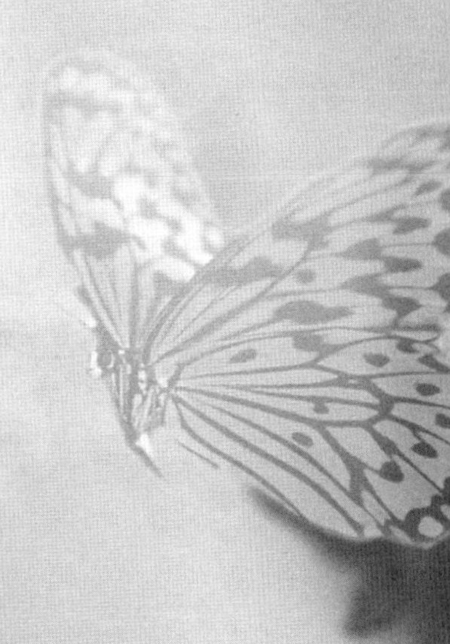

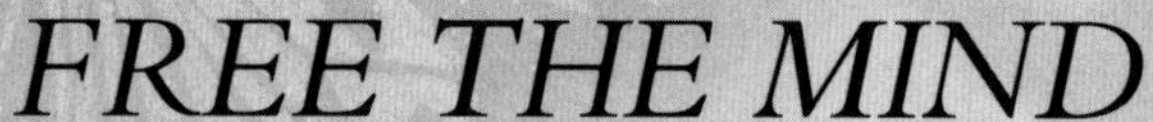

FREE THE MIND

I need to take my head off and hang it up.
I want the purity of cleansing air to free it of all sadness,
It is dark, but when the sun awakes
It will beam its golden rays into my clouded mind.

Kelly Howard, Year 11, Matthew Flinders GSC

(Published in the Living Poets Society –
So we bounced onto the moon, 1996)

CHAPTER 3
The Beginning of the End

Christmas 1999 was fun. The family gathered together at our place for lunch as usual, with some of the kids' friends joining us for tea. We set up the trestle tables on the decking; the weather was mild making for a pleasant Christmas afternoon.

Fiona and her partner Damian, Joshua and one year old Hayley came down mid-morning. Then, armed with glasses of champagne, Fiona, Kelly and I started cooking and setting the tables for lunch. Ross's parents – Marnie and Pa to everyone – were coming, along with the rest of his family. We would serve about 18 for lunch and each family contributed to the meal, so it was no big burden on us.

The boys set up the tables, and the rest of the family arrived just before we served lunch. Then it was present time. With much laughter, Pa donned his Santa hat, and enlisted the younger ones help to distribute the presents. It was a lovely day, with much merriment and no hint of the troubles that were to start early in the New Year.

New Year 2000 came and went; Kelly was the only one left living at home with us. She was in and out with her friends, driving her little car around, keeping busy. Not working in a job at that time, she had plenty of time on her hands.

The changes were quite subtle, so that we really didn't notice right away. Kelly spent a lot of time with Fiona, Damian and the children. She also caught up with Matt fairly regularly, but was mostly with her own friends. She had a boyfriend, Troy, with whom she also spent a lot of time.

Then Kelly moved out to live with Carolyn and Brad in Jan Juc for a while, and later to a little house up the road from us and around the corner from Fiona. Over the next few weeks, even though we saw her quite regularly, it was never for very long. She would just pop in, say hello and then be off again; so the signs of her deteriorating mental health were not obvious to Ross and me.

I was aware that she was smoking marijuana, but not the extent of it. Damian later made the comment that she was smoking quite heavily, but we were blissfully unaware that too much marijuana could potentially cause some psychological problems. When we realised that Kelly was having some problems, we still did not associate her behaviour with mental health issues. In fact, the words "mental health" were not even on the radar for us.

Kelly had secured a job in a small boutique in the city that specialised in recycled or second-hand clothing – a little more upmarket than an op shop – and she was so excited.

Doing very well initially, Kelly was really in her element working there. We were very happy that she had finally found a job, especially something she really enjoyed. It certainly suited her.

But then she started to "borrow" clothes and jewellery, leaving notes for the shop owner to say that she owed for this and that. She was busy making many little notes and lists, their meanings known only to Kelly.

She began carrying plastic bags of clothing around wherever she went, and we joked about her being a bag lady. Aside from that she seemed to be relatively OK. However, as we came to realise later, this was evidence of her deteriorating mental state.

Kelly arrived unexpectedly at Fiona and Damian's house early one Sunday morning. Telling them she'd run out of petrol, she asked if they could give her some. Damian gave her the mower fuel tin filled with petrol. Fiona and Damian were about to leave for a day in Melbourne and were running late. When they arrived in Melbourne, they discovered that Joshua had Kelly's car keys in his pocket.

Late that evening, Ross answered a knock on the front door to find the police there, asking if our car had been stolen. (Kelly's car was registered in my name.) It had been found just around the corner from Fiona's house with the bonnet up and parked rather haphazardly.

Ross and I drove up to collect it. We had to jump-start it to get it going. I got in to drive it home, but couldn't keep the engine running as it had run so dry of fuel.

This car had been Kelly's pride and joy when she first got it, and now the floor was littered with empty McDonald's wrappers, cut up pictures from magazines, empty drink bottles and junk jewellery from the shop – all of which had to inhibit safe driving practice. Ross ended up having to drive the car so I got in the passenger side. My knees were up under my chin because the rubbish was piled so high on the floor.

Fiona and Damian returned from Melbourne later that night to find Kelly asleep in their back room after she had broken into their house.

She had collected an odd assortment of groceries – a jar of peanut butter, a packet of couscous, a tin of tomatoes and a phone charger amongst other items – which were in a basket beside the front door. She'd also had a shower and helped herself to some of Fiona's clothes.

When asked about this, Kelly said she was going on a picnic (knowing she couldn't drive the car without petrol or key). Fiona and Damian talked to her until after midnight, and then Fiona drove her home to us. Kelly then came inside and phoned the Swanston Centre and arranged to be admitted. This was in mid-March 2000.

The Swanston Centre was the modern re-named Dax House psychiatric ward. We visited Kelly there, and she seemed quite comfortable and at ease. We spoke to her nurse, and we were invited to participate in a family meeting with the psychiatrist, to be convened at mutually agreeable time. They were very caring and kind to us.

Ross, Matthew, Fiona and I attended the Swanston Centre for the meeting with Kelly and the psychiatrist. We were shown to a small, rather cramped room, where the six of us crowded in. The meeting went well. We all had input and were treated with respect by the psychiatrist, Dr K. Kelly was able to put her viewpoints across, and everyone was listened to.

At the conclusion of the meeting, the psychiatrist said that he didn't know why Kelly was there, and that there was nothing wrong with her so she could go home. We left feeling relieved that all was OK, that Kelly was fine and that she was coming home.

But things didn't really change much over the next few weeks, which prompted me to write a letter to Kelly in an attempt to re-establish some meaningful communication.

Monday 10 April 2000

Dear Kelly,

I thought I would attempt to communicate with you via a letter, since it has been proven almost impossible to do so verbally lately. Dad and I have been through quite a range of emotions in the past few weeks – frustrated, angry, and not by any means least – concerned, to name but a few!

Last night you came home, walked in the door and said hello. Then, you disappear up to your room. Later you ask if you can cook tea. You cook up a large meal, eat a very small portion of it, leave most in the saucepan on the stove, and your dirty dishes in the sink.

Two weeks ago you made it *more* than clear at the Swanston Centre, that you (for reasons still unclear to us) could never live at home! Quite a change from the declaration of a few weeks before when you were going to stay living at home for at least the next three years because you could save lots of money living at home!

Last night, you seemed to be very busy in and around the house – up and down to your room, with not a word spoken to us. Your idea of doing the dishes was to put them in soapy water and leave them. You went outside, and I saw you get your purse.

Sometime later, when we wanted to go to bed and lock up the house, you were nowhere to be found. Dad went out and called to you but you didn't answer.

Now, as you no longer live here, we assumed that you had decided to go without saying good-bye, which is not unusual behaviour for you recently. We locked up and went to bed, only to find this morning that you have been back and exchanged bags after we went to bed.

Where were you? Why didn't you answer Dad when he called – it was dark and one can only wonder what on earth you were doing that you couldn't reply!

You surely must agree that you have exhibited some bizarre behaviour over these past weeks, and your whole family has been extremely concerned.

On the Tuesday at the Swanston Centre, you state that you couldn't possibly live at home anymore, then on the Wednesday you ring at 5 pm and leave a message that you are coming home that night. You arrive in the early hours of the morning, long after we have gone to bed, and you bring a "friend" home that we've never met, and play music loudly in your room and even burn a candle there! Then you get upset when I come up and demand to know who your "friend" is in bed with you! You are insolent when I ask you about the candle, and later upset when I ask for the key to the back door.

I think we are justified in being concerned about you having a key, when you show no respect for us and our property by burning a candle in your room – plus the room reeked of cigarette smoke.

We feel uncomfortable having you waltz in here anytime, with whoever when we are not here. By your own admission this is not your home anymore, and I believe we are within our rights to expect you to only come here when one of us is here.

The girl we have been seeing lately is not the Kelly we know and love; she is someone else inhabiting your body. But as much as we may wish to have our old Kelly back, we still love you, but unfortunately you haven't given us much reason to trust you of late.

When you refused to come back home to live, Catriona very kindly offered you a place to stay. We understand that you paid her rent, but she has rung up here quite concerned, as she hasn't seen you for several days. Claire has been ringing up looking for you, as she is also concerned because you have left your cases at her house. Now yesterday you talk about going to live at the River End Caravan Park – why?

Then there is the matter of the ute keys. Dad had searched for days for them as they held the only key to the petrol tank. It took some time for us to realise that you had taken them. Then when you admitted it on Friday night and said you would bring them back but didn't, we were more concerned.

You used those keys to get into the house on Thursday and do some washing, which incidentally is still sitting in the basket waiting to be hung out. Now we are not going to do that for you, as we remember your vehement avowal in that Tuesday meeting that you "**do your own washing!**"

For some reason, we – the family – seem to have become your enemies.

You sorted through the bag of clothes that Fiona kindly collected from the shop, and left the bag of smelly, wet washing (that was found on the floor of the shop!) here. Now it will probably have to be thrown out, as I doubt you will ever get the smell out of it, not to mention the mould that must be starting on it by now.

I could go on and on with anecdotes from the past few weeks, but I won't for now. Suffice to say that we, your family do love and care for you. We are all concerned with your strange behaviour, and would dearly love to be able to help you. Unfortunately, I believe that this time you may have to help yourself, as you have continually rejected our offers of help.

Love, as always, Mum & Dad.

I didn't actually get a response to this letter, but at least I felt better having expressed myself to her.

Then over the next few weeks, there were a series of disturbing events, which I documented in my journal.

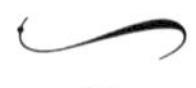

On the 26th April we wake to find Kelly has let herself into the house having stolen a key once again. She is asleep on a chair in the lounge. On a tray in front of the TV there is an open packet of biscuits, a bowl of dry noodles, a container of dip, Joshua's glass with some sort of drink in it, purses, manicure set, butterfly hairclip, a bank withdrawal slip, as well as the keys to Ross's work vehicle. There is a container of cut-up food and some veggie burgers sitting beside that near the stove. Beside the kitchen sink is the remaining rubbish from the cut-up food with a cigarette lighter sitting on top.

Outside she has been working on her car, in the backyard, which has been disabled (unbeknownst to Kelly). There is a large colourful sarong spread out neatly over the roof of the car, and a large piece of white taffeta is arranged in the shape of a bow on the back window. A wire pot-plant rack has been used to prop the boot open, and several windows have been left open, leaving the contents of the car very damp with dew.

She is wearing different clothes from when she left here last evening. When she was leaving, Ross had asked if she would be coming back and she said she wasn't.

She had come home yesterday around lunchtime, helping herself to food, then went into the front room, wandered in and out for a while, and then disappeared upstairs for several hours. We assumed she was sleeping.

That year the family headed off to the Forrest camping ground for our regular Easter get-together. We took the campervan and tents enough to house us all. Kelly didn't come, so we felt a little out of kilter with one family member missing, but we still had a good time.

We arrived home to find that Kelly had broken into the house again. This time she used a ladder, climbing onto the roof and letting herself in through the upstairs window. She has made it abundantly clear that this is no longer her home and that she could never live here again. So it's a puzzle why she keeps breaking in.

I asked what she had done for the weekend and she told me she'd had a lovely time with the Pollock family in Anglesea, who we had not heard of before. When I asked what day she came home, she said, "Oh, Friday or Saturday, I don't know, ask Pauline."

Pauline, our next-door neighbour had been feeding the animals whilst we were away. She said Kelly was there on Friday and she had a couple of blokes with her, and was home for virtually the whole weekend. Kelly had told Pauline that she'd gone to Melbourne, but was scared so she came home. She said she'd been kicked off the train at Werribee because she didn't have a ticket. A friend had then driven to Werribee to pick her up, but apparently wasn't very happy about it. We didn't know who this was.

Another neighbour, Susan, rang and spoke to her on Sunday evening and said that Kelly sounded really "out of it" and she thought she'd woken her up, but Kelly said no, she was unwell. Kelly also told Susan that she hadn't been invited to go camping with the rest of the family, nor was she welcome anywhere with us.

On the Thursday prior to Easter, Kelly had rung home and spoken to Ross who told her we were going camping and that we would very much like her to come with us. He said we would be leaving around 10.30 am on Friday and for her to be here by then if she wanted to come.

Kelly rang around midday on Friday and sounded sick and croaky and said she wasn't coming with us.

Susan rang again last evening while we were out and spoke to Kelly; she said once again Kelly sounded really "out of it". Susan apologised for waking her up again, but Kelly said that she hadn't been asleep, but she had conjunctivitis!

We went out for about an hour last evening, and when we returned Kelly wasn't there, but there was a mug on the bench with custard in it. Before we left, she said she had to pack her car because she had to find somewhere to live, and then before Ross could say any more, she said, "I know, you can't take the car, it's not roadworthy!"

Kelly also told Susan that she'd been keeping diaries for a long time, and that she's got one from grade one and even one from kindergarten. She also referred several times to the fact that Mum isn't handling "it" very well, which Susan understood to mean the sexual abuse. Susan felt she was talking to a totally different Kelly – something I've often felt, for quite some time.

Her room upstairs is an absolute mess. There are clothes strewn all over the floor, contents of bags and purses – of which she has many – are scattered haphazardly, making it difficult to step anywhere in the room without standing on something.

At the base of the stairs, is a pile of clothing and assorted possessions about 18 inches high and spread over an area of five to six feet. A laundry basket that had had her washing in it has now got some rubbish, a plastic bag with a half-full container of alfalfa sprouts, an open packet of dehydrated milk. Another basket has letters from a school friend, that to our knowledge, she hasn't had anything to do with for months. All of this is the absolute opposite of the Kelly we knew before Christmas. Kelly was our tidy one, always neat, and everything sorted and it its place. To see such a mess is quite upsetting.

Last night whilst we slept, Kelly has been looking around the house. She has drawn question marks on the notes I'd made whilst talking to Susan. Ross and I feel very vulnerable – almost violated because she has been so vehement and vocal with her attitude towards staying here, yet she continually breaks into the house and helps herself to food, goes through our things with a total disregard to our privacy. It is quite disturbing to know someone has been creeping around the house whilst we sleep. The Kelly of old would never have behaved like this.

A couple of weeks ago Kelly told Ross and I that she'd been asked by five different bands to sing for them, and that she was doing the make-up for several plays in town. She also told Susan on Sunday that she didn't need to have children as she's raised Joshua and Hayley herself.

Two weeks ago Kelly rang from Melbourne asking for her cousins' phone number. Later that night, around 10.15 p.m. she rang again, this time from Flinders Street Station in Melbourne, quite distressed because no-one would help her, and could I ring Teresa (her cousin) to say she was on her way. When I questioned her as to why she was in Melbourne, she hung up. I phoned her cousin Marcus to say she was on her way. When Kelly arrived not long after, they said she was quite calm with no evidence of the distress from our call. Marcus's girlfriend Mel said Kelly's foot was swollen up like a balloon, but either she couldn't remember or wouldn't say what she had done to it.

She stayed with her cousins for over a week. Marcus suggested she might be bulimic, as she eats a lot for someone so skinny. There was a bottle of toilet cleaner sitting on the floor beside the toilet, that hadn't moved for months, but when Kelly stayed there it was going from one side of the toilet to the other frequently. Marcus has had some dealings with eating disorders, as one of his sisters had required psychiatric treatment and hospitalisation for anorexia.

Whilst Kelly was with her cousins, she was very angry with us, and was telling them stories of our treatment of her. She said she was scared to go back to Geelong because "People want to kill me because I won't take drugs anymore".

She adamantly denied – without being asked – that she was on drugs, but on at least two occasions her cousins smelt marijuana and were fairly certain she was smoking it.

Kelly also told them that she couldn't read, and when it was pointed out to her that she'd just read something, she said that she couldn't read black and white, only colour. It was then noted that the passage she'd just read was black printing, and then Kelly told them that she could read any language put in front of her!

On the 19th April Mel took Kelly to Spencer Street Station and gave her $5 from her limited supply, as Kelly had said she had no money for her fare to Geelong. But much to Mel's dismay, Kelly went to Hungry Jacks and spent the money on food.

Later Kelly rang from the station and spoke to Ross; she was upset because she wanted to come home but had no money. When Ross asked if she had been given any money for her train fare (Marcus had called to say she was on her way), she became more upset and hung up. We contacted Spencer Street Station and asked them to page her for us, as we thought we may have been able to pay for her ticket at Geelong station, however she didn't answer the page.

Later she rang from a pizza shop in Spencer Street, and left a message asking us to call her back. I rang the shop and asked the woman who answered what sort of emotional state she was in, and she said she'd been upset but was fine now. Kelly spoke to Fiona and said the lady in the shop was nice and had given her some pizza and that she'd be home tomorrow. When Fiona asked how she was going to get home if she didn't have any money, she said she'd wash dishes or sing to earn some.

One evening last week, Susan and her children were visiting, and we decided to get takeaway for tea. Kelly made several phone calls, and said she was meeting Matt for a coffee at 6 pm however didn't make any real effort to get there, which made me think she was waiting for someone to offer to take her into town.

Many of the calls she was making were to mobile phones, so I commented that I'd be watching the next phone bill, as she'd be paying for some of these calls. Later Matt said she'd called him on his mobile three or four times, despite her assuring me they were only local calls.

Kelly then made a call in front of Susan and I, and loudly asked about reporting a sexual assault. She then told us she was being transferred to someone else and then repeated the story about a sexual assault she suffered by a train driver or conductor in Melbourne last week. Hanging up she said that the police were coming to take a statement, as they wouldn't do it over the phone. She also told Susan that she wouldn't make a scene in front of her children.

I went to collect tea, and Kelly was telling Susan – who is a former policewoman – about several sexual assaults over the past weeks. Sometime later, when no police had arrived, she made another phone call and cancelled the visit, but then proceeded to tell her story/statement over the phone. She appeared to be calling, but was pretending to do so.

She also called an old school friend, who she'd seen recently (her suitcase and some bags had been left at Claire's house.) Kelly then started to leave, and told us she was going to stay with Claire in Ocean Grove. When we asked how she was going to get there, she said she had lots of friends with cars who would drive her there, but could only name two when we asked whom they were. She said that Claire's family had gone away for the holidays, and she needed her to stay, as she was scared on her own.

Kelly changes clothes frequently, it is common to see her in four different outfits in an evening here. She has also been seen in a nightclub changing clothes and offering clothes to people. Another friend, Carolyn, said that Kelly had given her portable stereo to her. This is the same girl that Kelly didn't want to have anything to do with because "she's on drugs". Then a few weeks ago she called Matt and told him that Carolyn wanted to kill her, and that she had bashed Kelly up.

On the 28th April Kelly arrived home at 8.30 in the morning with two male friends we'd never seen before. I commented that I wasn't keen on visitors at that hour of the day. They didn't come inside with her, and she just collected some things, asked to use the phone, rang a taxi and they left.

The next day Kelly called Fiona and met her down the street, and then they both came home. I asked Kelly if she'd had any calls from Barwon Health. She said yes, and that Dr K, the psychiatrist wanted to see her. I asked if she was going to do that and she said she couldn't get in until May. I said that it was almost May, and she wouldn't have to wait very long. She then admitted she didn't want to see him, as she had lots of people helping her at the moment.

We talked some more, and then she got very upset, yelling that she'd have to grow up and that she was very, very sorry. She then went off, packed some bags and left with Fiona. Later Fiona brought the bags back home as Kelly had left them in her car.

That night, Fiona and Damian were still here. Ross and I had gone out when Kelly came home with her school friend Cara and a neighbour. She said Cara was going to help her jump-start her car, which wouldn't start because, unbeknownst to Kelly, Damian had removed the rotor button as the car wasn't safe for night driving. In addition, Kelly had had two minor accidents, and we were concerned that she wasn't safe to be driving. We worried that the next accident may seriously injure someone as she did not seem to be functioning very well mentally.

After her futile attempts to start the car, she left and later rang leaving a message here saying she was with Carolyn (the friend she said was trying to kill her) and wasn't feeling well, could we call her. She knew we had gone out for the evening.

When we got home, I didn't check the phone messages until late, then called Kelly and asked if she was all right. She said she was, and that she'd been with the neighbour who was calling her mother, and then Carolyn and her boyfriend walked past. Carolyn supposedly made some derogatory comments to Kelly. None of this conversation made sense, as she'd left a message saying that she was with Carolyn.

I looked through some of the bags lying at the bottom of the stairs. In one bag was what remained of a pair of jeans and a T-shirt that had been cut up into very small pieces, and smelt of stale urine? Another jumper had the sleeves cut off rendering it useless to wear. Most of the clothes were dirty, yet at the triage team meeting at the Swanston Centre on Wednesday, she'd insisted that they were clean and just needed ironing and folding.

30th April in the evening. Kelly called Fiona and spoke for around a quarter of an hour. The conversation was rather disjointed. She spoke of buying Matthew's car, and selling hers. Fiona suggested it would be cheaper to get her car fixed, and she agreed, saying, "Yes I know, that's what I'm going to do." She then told Fiona she was going to give her car to Sarah (whoever she is) because she is turning 18 and it will be a birthday present.

Fiona asked her where she was calling from, and she said "R's" – a former neighbour of ours that Kelly previously wasn't really comfortable with. When Fiona asked about the phone call and who was paying for it, Kelly said it was R's phone and it didn't matter. She also told Fiona she was working for BAYSA – a local youth support group. Fiona then asked how long she had been working for them and Kelly replied "Oh, since I bumped into Marcus and Mel the other week." (Kelly stayed with them in Melbourne until the 18th and this was the first we'd heard of her working for BAYSA.)

Kelly called me and asked how I was. Asked if I had the kids – she'd spoken to Fiona an hour before and was told that Hayley was in bed and Joshua in the bath. Then she said, "I've got the kids!" I asked whose kids, and how old are they? She said they are at BAYSA and they range from five days to 40 years. I said that you mustn't need any qualifications to do that, and she said she is just helping out, that they are all her age, if not older or younger!

Also she had some mattresses, cigarettes and food to deliver to people, and she was coming around to get her car so she could do that. Then she said that there are people there who can fix her car for nothing, and she was going to sell her car to a friend, for his girlfriend Sarah. When I enquired how much for, she said she didn't know.

Then she said she needed to get another car – one without a gearbox – an automatic. She thought she would get this new car and have gas put on because she is not made of money. I said she would need a lot of money to do all she wants, and Kelly said that all these people are going to help her for free.

I asked her again about going to the hospital to get checked out, and she said yes, she was going to do that, that she was "Going to see all my little psych nurse friends, because they practise their blood pressure and things on me." And "I teach them, and we are learning together. They are my friends." She then said she had to go because this was not her phone.

WHY?

Sometimes I wonder …
What do you think?
Why do you think about...?
How do you feel?
Why do you run?
Why do you hide?
Why do you close up?
Why not stop?
Why not open?
Why do you not stand?
Why is there confusion?
Why is there selfishness?
Why is the grass dead?
Why is your sky grey?
How much time do you need?
When will you heal?
How deep is your pain?
When will you shed your fear?
Are you scared?
Are you sick?
Are you impatient?
Are you sad?
Have you enough strength?

Why not drop your barrier?
Have you no time?
I thought, I worried, tried.
I understood, I knew.
I closed, I opened, I cried.
I fell, I waited, I will see.
I think.
Are you cold?
Do you wonder?
Do you see?
Do you want?
Can you reach?
You know,
I know,
You know,
You need.
You're going to stop.
You're going to fall.
You are falling.
Will you be caught?
Are your tears hiding it all?
What will it take?
When will you realise?
Why not see the hurt you deal?
Why not prove yourself to yourself?
Why not focus on that?
Why not focus?

Fiona Howard, 17 April 2000

CHAPTER 4

The Continuing Slide

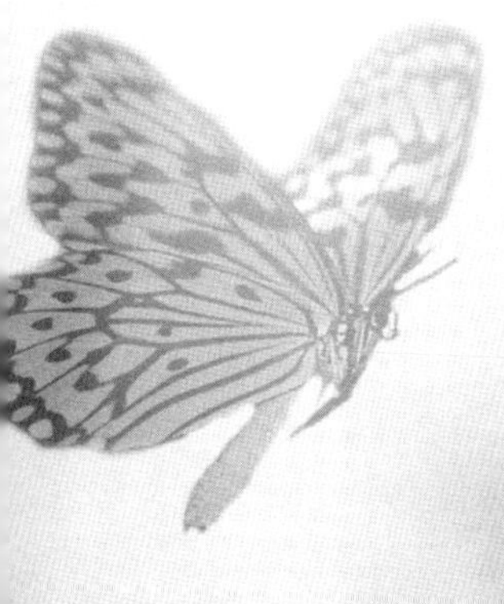

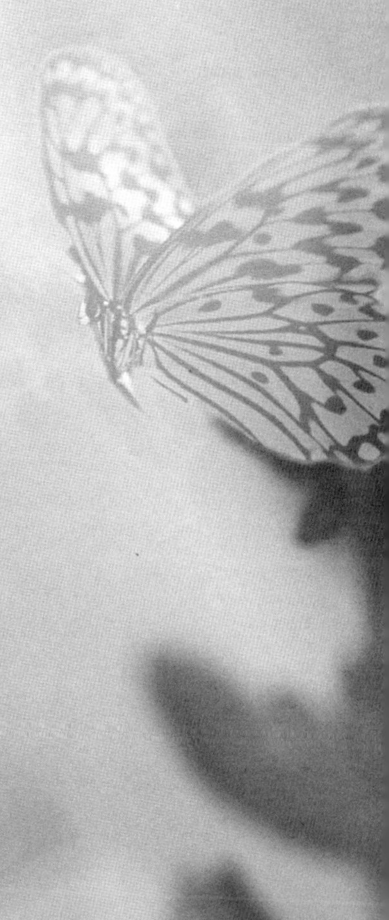

FEAR

I'm so afraid
I know I am
Tonight I cry
I'm a living volcano
Nothing's changed
No-one knows me
No-one
I mask my emotions
My life
I breathe
Because I think I want to.

Kelly Howard, 1999

CHAPTER 4
The Continuing Slide

1 May 2000

Kelly called into home around 7 pm; said she had friends waiting in the car so couldn't stay long, and had just come to get some schoolbooks to sell to a friend. Whilst here, she changed into some extra clothing – a woolen jumper, followed by another cotton one over the top and inside out. She seemed fine, perhaps a little over the top but not manic.

***

2 May 2000

I received a call from Kelly at 10 am, saying she was at the hospital accident and emergency (A & E), waiting to see a doctor. She said she'd been to all the medical clinics and no one would keep a place for her, so she had to wait. She said she needed her school books, plus some milk and bread because she had to give them to some people. Also she needed money to pay people back for petrol and board. I said I might come in later.

When Kelly hung up, I called A & E and asked to speak to the nurse in charge. I explained the situation with Kelly, and asked her to call the psych triage team to assess her whilst she was there.

Kelly phoned again around 11 am; said she'd finished at A & E, and she'd seen the same guy from psych triage last Wednesday. She then asked if I was going to pick her up and that she could meet me at McDonalds in the city.

I met Kelly at McDonalds, bought her a Happy Meal and had a coffee with her. It was difficult to watch her eating a Happy Meal that included meat, as she had been a vegetarian for several years. I'd noted a lot of McDonalds wrappers in the rubbish on the floor of her car, so she'd been eating meat for some time.

We talked for a while and then I asked her a few pointed questions about "R" – a former neighbour who worked at BAYSA. Matthew said he'd spoken to R last evening and that she'd said Kelly had been very good, and that "She's only had one gram of marijuana since last Friday!" Kelly got upset at this denying that she'd had any.

I asked her why she'd involved R, because I am upset that this woman feels she can lecture my family on our problems when she can't even handle her own family issues.

Kelly cried then, and said she had to go back to the hospital to get her referral to see the doctor. I said I thought she'd finished there. We got in the car and drove back to the Swanston Centre. We were shown into the triage team office, where Jerome and another nurse interviewed Kelly.

Later Jerome showed Kelly the back way to A & E. He told me that whilst they would like to admit Kelly, unless she volunteers to be admitted, they can't do anything if she decides to walk out. She really needs medication and a stay of at least two days there. I said I would try and talk her into it, but wasn't too confident of my success.

I left to go and get Kelly from A & E, but she wasn't there. The nurse told me she had gone to try and find a smoke. I went outside to look but couldn't see her. I went back in to tell the staff that I'd gone to the gym when Kelly returned. She had apparently met Catriona (Quill's mother) outside pathology and they'd been talking. So we sat in the waiting room and I asked her why she was there, what was wrong? Kelly said she wanted blood tests for vitamins; her blood pressure taken and to be weighed; then she said, "I tell them I'm pregnant so they will do the tests, and maybe a urine test too!"

I suggested that perhaps she was wasting their time and she agreed with me. So we got up and walked outside. I said that if she wanted my opinion, then I felt she needed help emotionally and that the best place to help her was the Swanston Centre. We walked back around the block, and talked.

Kelly says she has a "fear" of uniforms on trains etc. because of what happened in Melbourne. Perhaps something did happen, but because so much of what Kelly has been saying has not made any sense, none of us have believed her. Kelly also said that she was made to look like a fool because she is still waiting for the police to contact her. I asked if she had actually been to the police station, and she said she'd been past it lots of times, but not gone in. I suggested she needed to actually go in and make a complaint.

Kelly then said she would like to go and see her cousin in Adelaide, but that no one would give her Stacey's address. Then, "She's probably on drugs too!" I asked why she should be and Kelly replied, "Why wouldn't any of my cousins be on drugs?" (Inferring, I assume because of my father's actions). Then, Kelly said she would have to sit down because she was feeling weak, as she hadn't eaten. Surprised, I said, "But I just bought you a Happy Meal!" and she said, "That wasn't food!"

Then she cried and said she was scared of Rob – R's boyfriend. He yells at her all the time, and she'd have to take bread, milk and chocolate to him when she goes back. I asked why she goes back if she's scared of him, and she said because she has nowhere else to go. Then she said she is really clean, although she can't have a shower because she can't stand for very long and she is the cleanest person she knows as she washes every other day!

We stood talking outside the Swanston Centre for quite a while, until finally she said she would stay. She also said she wanted a drink, so I agreed to buy her one. As we walked down the drive towards the Centre, I asked her a couple of times if she meant it, and she said yes. Once there, I bought her a Coke and a chocolate bar from the vending machine and Kelly gave me her phone because it was almost out of credit (people keep using her phone and using up all her credit she said). She also gave me a slip for photo collection and another for a lay-by she had put aside.

Jerome came and took us inside, and then Kelly changed her mind and decided she wouldn't stay. Dismayed, I said, "But you told me you would!" I think she only said that so I'd buy her a drink.

I told Jerome that I'd suggested she was wasting time at A & E, and he agreed. He asked Kelly if she would consider coming in and having her tests done whilst she was in there. She said no. Then she said she would talk to Janette M – another psychiatrist. So Jerome rang and made an appointment for her on Thursday at two o'clock. Now we just have to get her there.

We were still talking when Kelly said, "When I go nightclubbing, I see my psych nurse friends and they take my blood pressure, they practise on me and I learn and they learn too, it's fun!" Jerome and I looked at each other and raised our eyebrows in silent communication.

We then left after making a joke with Jerome about Kelly not taking him up on his repeated offers of hospitality. At the car Kelly said she really needed a smoke, a jerry can with five dollars of petrol, plus some bread and milk. I then took her to the 7-Eleven and bought her cigarettes. Then I drove to the gym, parked and told Kelly I was going in. I gave her ten cigarettes, so that no-one could scam them off her and handed over five dollars and she left.

Later I met Matt and Quill for a coffee and we talked. Matthew was upset because Kelly was going to have coffee with them and Fiona last night, but after having several phone conversations with her, they realised she wasn't coming. First she said she was just leaving Clonard Avenue, and then she said she had to go to Albert Street to pick something up, and then next call R answered. She then proceeded to lecture him on the problems of the family and so on. Then she asked him if I was still on holidays and if he would set up a time for her to talk to me. Matthew said that there was really no need for her to get involved. Later he had more calls from her but he didn't answer them.

When Matt and I were walking back to the car, Kelly called Matt and asked if I was with him, and could I call her at Brooke's house. So when I got home I tried ringing the number but it was engaged. Ross got the messages off our phone, and there was one from Kelly saying she would be at Catriona's until six o'clock. I rang Catriona, Kelly wasn't there, but might be coming for tea.

Then Kelly rang home and was rather upset with me, as she wanted her smokes and her phone. She asked me to drive to Weller Street – around the corner – and pick her up. I asked why she couldn't just walk around to us, which upset her even more and she hung up. She then called Ross on his mobile but I answered it. She said she wanted to talk to him not me but hung up again.

Later Fiona arrived with Kelly and a guy she had met at the Swanston Centre when she was an inpatient.

Kelly gets upset with me very quickly, most likely because I challenge some of her rather questionable statements. She starts talking about something and then goes off on another tangent, so it is difficult at times to make sense of what she is saying.

She asked me for her phone, and I reminded her that she had given it to me to use, but I said she could have it back. She then tried to give it back to me. I hadn't used it, nor put any credit on it. She talked again of going back to school to complete Year 12 as she had finished all her CATs (Common Assessment Tasks) – but I said she hadn't and she got upset again and started yelling at me.

They left with Fiona, who rang me later and said she'd taken them to Clonard Avenue to see R, who was asking why I wanted Kelly to go to the Swanston Centre. Then R said she could take her, and Fiona replied, "So could I."

She then suggested that Kelly may have schizophrenia and Fiona responded, saying that you really couldn't make a diagnosis that easily as it could be any number of things similar. (I had printed information on schizophrenia off the net that Fiona had read, so she was glad she'd seen that before talking to her.) Fiona also said that there was no need for her to get involved in our family business. Fiona then took Kelly and her friend to Catriona's.

When Fiona returned home, she found Kelly's beautiful deb dress wrapped up in a T-shirt in her car. There was also another bag of smelly clothes; I said to bring them here so that I could wash them.

***

3rd May 2000

Kelly rang home just after lunch and asked what I was doing, did I have any plans and had I just got up! I replied that I wasn't doing anything in particular, as I am loath telling her exactly what I am doing or going to do. I said that I had someone to see in about 20 minutes.

She said she wanted to bring some friends around to help her fix her car. I asked who these friends were, and she said, "One is a girl." I commented that I didn't think she would be much help and Kelly got cross with me again. Kelly then said that this girl needed to go home, and I asked where she lived. Kelly replied "Geelong West". I asked why she needed the car fixed so she could go home, as we were already in Geelong West, and Kelly got cross again.

Kelly commented that school was nearly out. I asked what she meant by that, as she doesn't go to school anymore and Kelly said she wished she were.

Then she asked if I had her phone turned on, and I said I didn't. Kelly then asked me to turn it on as there were lots of messages on it, and she wanted it back as well as some smokes. I said I would leave the phone and the smokes on the outside table when I went out, which I did, but she didn't collect them.

Ross came home after work and said that Kelly had called him whilst he was working, asking to speak to Damian. Ross told her he was working with the snipper at the time, so Kelly said she wanted us to go to the Railway Hotel at six o'clock that night to hear her sing. She told him it was free, and that we just had to pay for our meal and drinks.

Ross and I have begun to doubt everything Kelly says now, it all seems so far-fetched. So we didn't believe that Kelly was really singing at the Railway Hotel. We chose to go out for dinner anyway, as we needed a break from the constant calls, arguments and stories. It was becoming very emotionally draining.

Once home, Kelly rang, saying she'd been around and collected three cigarettes! Then she asked if she could have $10 tomorrow – or $50 *because she owes people money for rent, or she could just come and write a cheque for $50. I said she couldn't write a cheque, as it would bounce, as she is not a signatory on the account anymore. Kelly then argued, yelling, "It's not fair. What have you ever done for the business? I've done a lot – more than you've ever done!"*

I asked why she thought she could just waltz in and write out a cheque, to which she replied, "Just shows what trust you have in me, I feel like a fucking idiot now!" Then she hung up the phone.

THIS IS ME

I know that I haven't achieved anything
But now I do realise,
That I myself am an individual
This is me, this is who I am!

Kelly Howard, 7 July 1995

CHAPTER 5

Conflict and Chaos

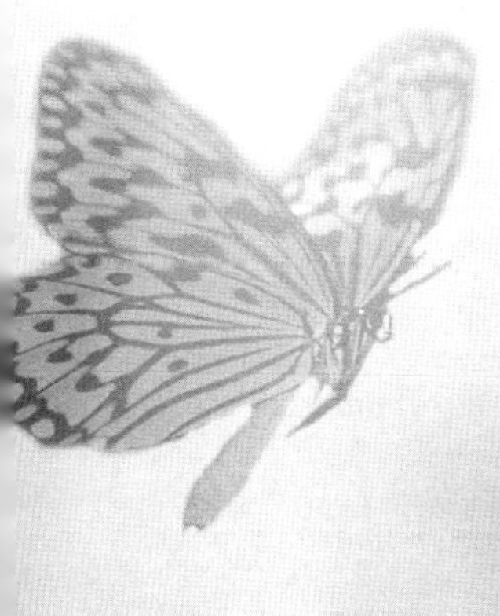

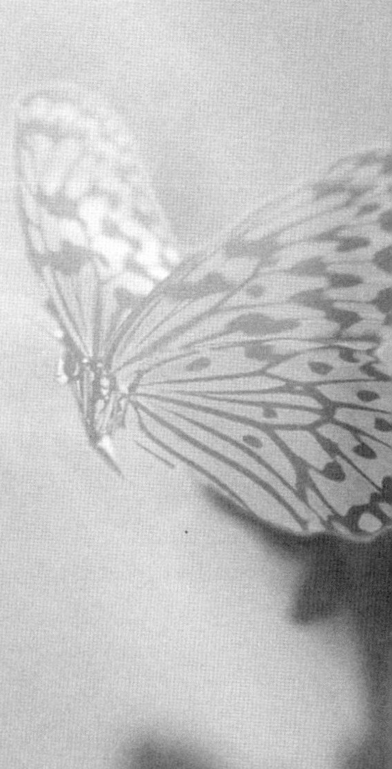

I FEAR NOTHING

You can shovel me up and whisk me away with your spade,
But I'm not going to be afraid.
You can come from behind and scare me whilst under shade.
But I'm not going to be afraid.
You can take away my soul to keep and have it remade,
But I'm not going to be afraid.
You can harm me by pulling the pin on your grenade.
But I'm not going to be afraid.
I fear nothing...

Kelly Howard, 12 November 1995

CHAPTER 5
Conflict and Chaos

4 May 2000

Kelly called at 10 am sounding terrible. Said she was really, really scared. Someone had left a threatening phone message yesterday. She asked if I could come and get her, as she had an appointment at 2 pm with Janette, the psychiatrist. I said Fiona was due here shortly, and we'd come and get her. Kelly called again at 10.30 am, sounding more aggressive and disgruntled.

When Fiona came we drove around to pick her up (about three blocks from home). She came out of the house with her usual assortment of bags, a couple of colourful ones stuffed full of clothes, and a man she introduced as Adam, who she had to get to school. I said we'd drop him off, and then she directed me to R's house, where she collected another bag of goods.

Kelly has bits and pieces of her belongings spread around Geelong at various places. I don't think she even remembers what she's got and where. After dropping Adam off at the Gordon, we came home around 11 am. Ross and Damian were still here, as Ross wanted to see Kelly before he went to work.

Kelly was meant to attend an appointment that morning with Anita from the Community Resource Centre, who was helping her find a job. I'd phoned earlier and explained that Kelly wasn't available. Anita returned my call, spoke to Kelly and gave her a name of someone who would help her with a job. She also had information on the STD clinic. Kelly seems obsessed with having blood tests for vitamins and checking for STDs.

Kelly then called R and invited her around to talk with me, as she is the only one who understands her, none of the family believes her.

We had lunch, and Kelly started packing up talking about a photo shoot to organise: she's doing the make-up; a gig to organise and an appointment with someone else this morning. It was almost noon.

I'd earlier removed the key from the security door so she couldn't leave that way, and I'd tied up the bolt on the side gate. Kelly prowled around the house, packing bags, going out to check her car, and then back to the kitchen for more food.

She went into the children's room and was packing and unpacking bags. She had a purse with her calisthenics medals in it, and said she was teaching children calisthenics – children whose parents couldn't afford to pay and parents who don't care about their children. These children love her.

Her behaviour became more erratic and manic. She said she needed to eat and I said you've just eaten, to which she replied, "That's not food!"

Then for the next half an hour Kelly was putting her bags on her bike and attempting to leave via the side gate. Fiona or I would stop her, as we were determined she see the psychiatrist.

Then she threw her bags over the gate, picked up her bike – I thought she was going to throw it at me! I took hold of her wrist, and although she tried to get away, she didn't really try very hard.

I led her back inside, and said to Fiona, "Even though it's only 1.30 pm, I think we will go, as I don't think it will matter if we are early." I felt it would be better there as it was getting very hard to take, her prowling around, trying to escape and abusing us.

Going inside I collected my bag and car keys, when Fiona rushed in to say she'd got away. Seizing a window of opportunity, Kelly quickly went around the side of the house. Her mountain bike was leaning against the fence, and because the gate was locked, with superhuman strength, she picked up the bike and threw it over the gate. Quite a feat as she was not very tall and the gate was over six foot high and the bike was rather heavy – I don't think I could have done it. Then she climbed over the gate, got on her bike and made her escape.

Fiona and I raced to my car and set out to find her. We drove around the surrounding streets, and eventually spotted her. Riding down a small incline coming towards us, and as she came closer we could see the look of absolute glee on her face, she put her hand up, gave us the finger and then waved! My window was down and as Kelly rode past she let out a loud "Wheee". It was funny really, but sad too. She was like a small child running away from the adults.

Eventually we caught up with her and were able to take her to the appointment with Janette, she came willingly and quite calmly – Fiona and I heaving great sighs of relief as we finally reached the waiting room.

The receptionist asked if there was anything Kelly needed, and she asked if she could take her blood pressure. So Karen took her blood pressure, Kelly said her arm was sore and swollen where Fiona had grabbed it. There were no marks nor was it swollen – and Karen agreed looking to pacify her.

Janette arrived saying she only had twenty minutes, and could we wait outside. Half an hour later, Janette called us in and explained that Kelly had agreed to let me get her script if she wrote a request for blood tests. She had also given Kelly a sample pack of tablets, telling her they were to help her sleep and some were to calm her down.

Kelly and I had sniped a bit at each other during the meeting, and Janette suggested we should keep apart because of it. It seemed a little unfair because I had been very controlled most of the time around Kelly, but was reaching the end of my tether. When Kelly left the room, Janette said that we have to try the tablets, but she didn't really believe Kelly would take them. The "sleeping" pills were anti-psychotics, and Janette said if she didn't cooperate this week, then she would probably have to certify her. I cried a little then and Janette gave me a hug, saying I should call her later to talk more. When I left, Kelly had already gone.

Later, when I had collected the tablets, I spotted Kelly in the main street, but she turned away pretending she hadn't seen me. I suggested to Fiona that they stay for tea, and we invited Matt and Quill too. I was dishing up tea when Kelly rang and asked if there was enough for her too. She rode here on her bike, and was here in a few minutes.

It was lovely having the whole family around the table on the decking, enjoying a meal together and a glass or two of wine. Then Fiona took offence at a derogatory comment Kelly made about Ross and I. Plates and glasses went flying, my wine was tipped over me, as Fiona and Kelly rolled around amid broken glass on the decking, brawling.

Damian and Matthew separated them and we sat down to talk again. Fiona had cut her toe, plus scraped her arm. Ross suggested that perhaps Kelly needed to go to the Swanston Centre again, for a little while, to get some help. Eventually agreeing, Ross said he would drive her in, and I was to phone them to let them know she was coming.

They left and I duly made the phone call. On the way into town, Kelly decided she didn't need to go. Ross reminded her that she had promised us, and urged her to co-operate.

When they arrived, Ross sat in the waiting room whilst Kelly was being interviewed. Janette, who was just leaving after her rounds, spotted Ross, and said, "Ross! What are you doing here?" When he explained, she said, "Leave it with me." Janette went back into the Centre, and shortly after Kelly was admitted as an involuntary patient.

The next morning I rang the Swanston Centre and spoke to Michael, Kelly's nurse for the day. He said Kelly was still sleeping and that he would call me later.

Around 11 am I received call from a very irate Kelly, who didn't want to talk to me but demanded her Dad. She then yelled at Ross for not bringing her any smokes.

I then called Michael, who said she'd been very "chaotic" in her actions. He'd heard her yelling at us on the phone. She'd seen Dr K the psychiatrist and one minute she'd be talking to him and the next she was talking to me, even though I wasn't there!

It was explained to her that she was an involuntary patient, and that she was unable to leave the building. Michael said the alternative was full lockdown, which can be very traumatic and she didn't warrant that. We discussed bringing in a couple of changes of clothes, smokes, toiletries and food, and I said I'd be in around 2 pm.

Fiona and I spent quite a bit of time going through some of Kelly's things, sorting out dirty laundry and rubbish – of which there is a lot. Then Fiona and I went into the Swanston Centre to visit Kelly. She was a little aggressive and asked if I had gone through her things. When I said yes, she asked if I'd read anything and I said no.

She showed us into her room – a double, and I was surprised to see how many of her bags she'd managed to bring with her. She really was such a bag lady. She then proceeded to put on some of the clothes I'd brought in.

Wearing her swimsuit as undies, she added a skirt I'd made for her a few months ago, which almost fell off because she's lost so much weight. Already wearing three tops, she put on another two, then made a trip to the bathroom and put on jeans beneath the skirt. She came out and said sarcastically, "Thanks Mum for washing these jeans, I've just found 50 bucks in the pocket and it's mine!" Later we swapped the $50 for a $20 as there was less chance of her losing that.

I spoke to Michael, who said she'd be kept in over the weekend for observation and he introduced me to her evening nurse. Kelly was scheduled to see Dr K on Monday for assessment, as it was too early to make a diagnosis. Fiona commented that she should write a book whilst she is in, and Kelly said, "Oh I have already, and made a movie, now I just have to put them together."

This stay in the Swanston Centre was vastly different to the previous one. On the Saturday Kelly phoned and left two messages, and when I returned the calls she was rather belligerent.

Later that evening Ross and I visited her and were left to trail along behind her whilst she totally ignored us. We watched her play a game of pool with another patient, and then we went into the piano room where we had to ask her to repeat anything she said, as the music was so loud. Following her out of there we stayed in the hallway looking at a painting, I remarked, "I wonder how long before she realises we're not behind her." Kelly came back to find us and asked if we were going and I said, "I don't think we are needed here, so yes, we probably will go."

She then started yelling at us. "I'm fucking bored shitless in here." Her language was very bad, so Ross turned and left. I went to the desk to let the nurses know that we were leaving as Kelly was upset, and the nurse commented that yes, she seemed a bit aggro as they'd heard her yelling at us. She also said they were aware that Kelly is rather volatile at the moment.

Ross was really angry at her language, he said he didn't care how sick she was and he felt there was no need for her to carry on like that.

Neither of us wanted to go back again with the way Kelly was behaving. It was so hard to take.

Sunday, Kelly rang to apologise, and I suggested that she would be better apologising to her father, which she did.

Monday Kelly rang us requesting her flute and music books, as well as her phone.

Later I spoke to her nurse, who said she is to stay possibly until the end of the week, and that there was to be a family meeting on Wednesday at 11 am. No diagnosis has been made, but we could ask then; she is also seeing Janette tomorrow.

Fiona, Hayley and I visited her, and she seemed pleased to see us. Kelly asked if I knew the charge nurse, and when I said no, she said, "She's picking on me – I can't do anything right!"

That evening Kelly rang and wanted to know why Fiona or Matthew weren't there with her, as "Fiona swung the first punch, and I could tell tales about Matt, and any number of people could be in here partying with me!" I said that she'd been behaving rather strangely of late, but Kelly seemed to think there was nothing wrong, and she doesn't know why she is there.

The next day was much the same, with phone calls from Kelly, alternating between aggression and crying, then pleading and hanging up on us. When we visited she had three friends I'd never met before with her and they seemed nice. After they left we went to her room and Kelly sat on the bed and talked/cried/talked. She said she didn't want to be in there, so I replied that she'd been behaving rather weirdly lately, and that she was there to find out what was wrong. Kelly said, "I know what is wrong!" but wouldn't tell us as "You don't listen and I've already told you."

On the Wednesday morning, Ross, Matthew, Fiona and I were shown into a large meeting room. Shortly after, a number of nursing staff started coming into the room and took up seats along the sides of the room. It felt like there was going to be a show of some sort, and we were the attraction!

The psychiatrist came in and sat in an armchair at the front of the room, and then Kelly marched in holding a clipboard. She was dressed nicely, and also sat at the front of the room.

At no time were we asked if we minded the others being there, it seemed that we didn't matter at all. I think there would have been easily twenty people, ready for the event.

Dr K started the meeting, gave his version of the facts, and then asked if we had anything to say. I responded, saying that I had made some notes about Kelly's behaviour over the past weeks and he said, "Share them then."

I stood and read out several pages outlining the bizarre behaviour of the past weeks.

When I'd finished, Dr K turned to Kelly and asked her for an explanation. Kelly gave a rather garbled account that didn't make much sense at all. Dr K then turned to me and said, "There you go, she was drunk!"

I was shocked, but there was no chance of a response.

Kelly went on to say that "Mum's the one with the issues here, she's the one with the problems!"

We had mentioned Kelly's erratic driving, and that we'd disabled the car so she couldn't drive it and injure someone. Dr K then said, "Fix it. Let her drive, she is an adult and the responsibility is hers."

Then, once again, "I don't know what she's doing here, there is nothing wrong with her! She can go home." We were stunned, but that was the end of the meeting. The onlookers filed out and we followed.

I was angry and hurt that no-one (Ross, Matthew or Fiona) had made any attempt to defend me. I felt like I'd been treated as a naughty schoolgirl, and that I was being chastised. I was also amazed to hear Dr K say that he didn't know why Kelly was there as there was nothing wrong with her. To me it wasn't normal to be having a conversation with someone who was not in the room, as Kelly had with him on the first morning of her stay.

We had to wait for Kelly to be discharged, and then took her home with us, where she stayed for a short time before leaving again. Needless to say the rotor button was not replaced on the car, as Ross felt Kelly was incapable of making rational decisions whilst driving, and would most likely have another accident.

I was still feeling used and abused, and I was angry that Ross was happy to have Kelly return home to live as if nothing had happened. I felt that my feelings were of little importance and I was hurt.

It took me some time to accept that Kelly had changed, and was nothing like the scattered, angry girl from the Swanston Centre. I suppose I was sulking a bit, having put so much effort into trying to get help for Kelly, and then being told there was nothing wrong.

To this day I struggle with that interpretation from a skilled professional who was meant to be there to help, but seemed not to care about the patient.

WORDS UNSPOKEN

The words I want to say are truly unclear.
So therefore, if spoken, will not rightly be heard.
I need to speak up and be comforted from my jumbled mind.
But who will listen and help me to uncover the falsified truth?
Within everyone's own mind, they speak an unspoken language.
And even when these words are spoken aloud, they are often misinterpreted and confused by another one's clouded mind.
Who is to judge these things?
Is there a way to convert one's thoughts and feelings into the evil eye of reality?
And if so, who is the bearer of the final say?

Kelly Howard, 14 July 1996

CHAPTER 6

The Final Day

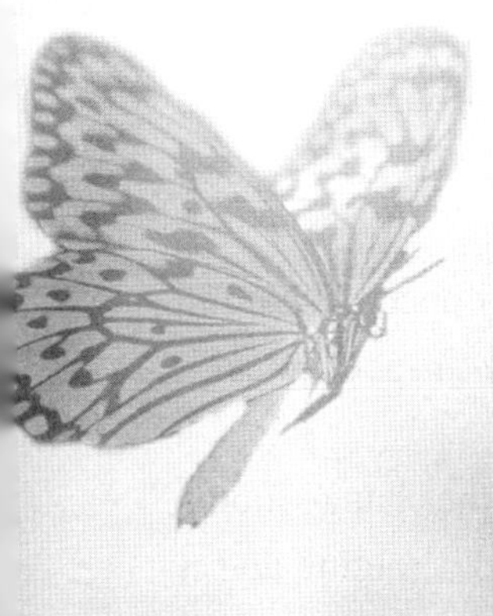

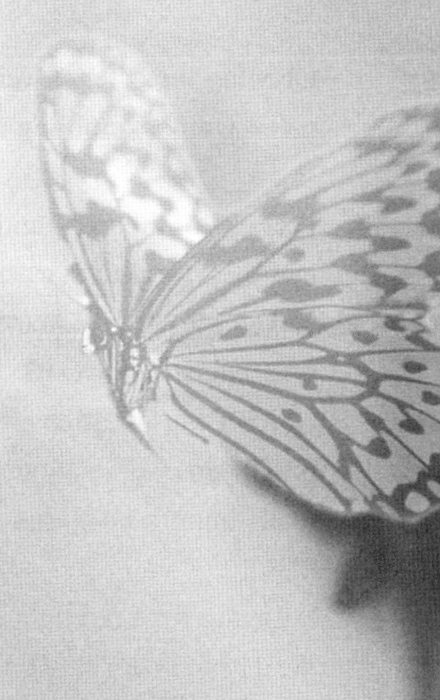

CHAPTER 6
The Final Day

The insistent buzz of the alarm woke me at 5.45 am. Groaning, I rolled over hitting the snooze button. My gear was packed and ready; I just had to pull on my gym clothes, wash my face and then hop in the car.

It was very dark at that hour of the morning in August, and cold, and I was glad I had my warm coat on. I didn't turn on the outside light, confident I knew the way across the decking to the carport and to the gate. I was the only one up – even the dog was still in bed!

Opening the gates, I went to the car and backed out, stopped to shut the gates again, grumbling under my breath about "bloody tin-pot" gates.

I set off for the gym, and once there, parked my bag in the change rooms and then went to start my usual circuit. I'd established a routine and it served me well. When finished I headed for the shower, and then got dressed ready for work. I finished getting ready except for my make-up, which I put on after breakfast at home. Breakfast, mmm! I fantasised on my way home about my porridge, thinking I couldn't wait, as I was really hungry now after that work-out.

Stopping for a red light, I reflected on last evening with Ross and Kelly. We'd watched *The Footy Show* and shared some laughs. Ross and I decided to get tickets for the live show in Melbourne next month, so I went online and ordered them. Kelly seemed to be enjoying herself.

It felt strange, having her at home again. She'd come back the week before, and had been rather quiet. I was still a little hesitant about her being there, but Ross was very encouraging so I'd gone along with him.

I suppose I still felt a little hurt after all the crap and weird stuff we'd been through over the past months, but she seemed to have put all that behind her. In fact you'd never guess that she'd had periods of extreme behaviour and irrationality. It was as if she'd never been gone, and I was starting feel that we were getting our Kelly back at last, the one we had last Christmas.

Because it was a weeknight I'd said my goodnights and gone off to bed before the show finished, closing the bedroom door to keep any television noise out. Not long after I heard Kelly's footsteps coming up the passage. She stopped outside my door for a while, and I was expecting her to knock and come in, but she left without a word.

Almost home now, and following my habit I turned up the side street that would bring me to the street in front of the house. I usually park out front as I will be off again in a little while and I don't have to battle with those gates again.

Reaching the T-intersection I stopped before turning right, when I noticed two ambulances parked in front of the house. I was also surprised to see two police cars there as well. There were other unfamiliar vehicles parked along the street. The bus had stopped across the road, and I initially think that someone has been hit.

Parking a couple of doors up the street, I grabbed my bag and started walking to the gate. The bus moved off. Then with a feeling of dread,

I began running through scenarios in my head. Had Ross had a heart attack? Or had something happened to Kelly? Then I noticed my front door was open so it definitely meant they're at my house. Walking up the path my mind was racing, my stomach in knots. What would I find inside?

I stepped through the open door, trembling now as I saw at the end of the passage men in blue crouched around a body on the floor. I started walking towards them and about halfway down the passage another man in blue appeared before me, asking, "Are you Mum?" I answered, "Yes, what's happened?" Still looking at the scene before me, I heard his reply. "I'm sorry, but your daughter's hung herself."

I took a deep breath and immediately morphed into charge nurse Howard and, squaring my shoulders, continued down towards the tragic scene at the end of the passage.

As I entered the room, the ambulance man at Kelly's head, who was squeezing the ventilator, looked up at me. I saw his dismay as he recognised me – he brought patients into work regularly and knew me quite well. I looked at him, raised an eyebrow in question and he sadly shook his head. I knew there was no hope now.

All this happened in a matter of seconds. I continued to my right, into the kitchen, and Ross spotted me. He reached for me crying, "Oh Chrissie!" and grabbed hold of me, sobbing and clutching me tightly. I returned the embrace, with tears slipping down my face. He was dragging me down, I couldn't move, and I was still wearing my coat. I held him for a moment, and then gently asked him to let me go so I could take it off. Then we clutched each other, rocking and crying together for what seemed like an eternity, but was probably only a few minutes.

Then another ambulance man came up to me, and asked me if I would come outside with him. I let Ross go and followed him outside onto the decking, stepping around the two men in blue working on Kelly's lifeless body, performing CPR, going through the motions.

Once outside, he said to me, "I'm sorry, but there is no response, so we need to stop the resuscitation." I nodded in agreement, having known from the outset that there was no hope, but that they were doing what they had to do.

He also asked if they could put her on her bed. I said, "But her bedroom's upstairs!" and he then asked about somewhere downstairs. So I took him to the spare room and showed him the bed there.

Then I returned to Ross in the kitchen. I said to him, "I'm going to get us a Valium each, as I think we'll need them." I went to the bedroom to get the Valium and one of us took one – I found the other one on the bench later, but couldn't say who didn't take it.

There was a policeman and a detective in the kitchen, and one of them asked me if I could show him Kelly's bedroom, as they needed to look for a note, or, as I realise later, to see if there were any signs of struggle, as they had to rule out homicide. It hadn't occurred to me that we might be considered suspects, but they were also just doing their job.

The detective took Ross outside and the policeman and I climbed the spiral staircase to Kelly's bedroom. Her bed was unmade, with only Pink Teddy there to tell the story and no sign of a note.

Coming back down the stairs, the policeman said to me, "You must be the strong one." I said, "No, it would be whoever was at home." Reaching the kitchen, he offered to make us a cup of tea.

I talked to the policeman about letting Matthew and Fiona know. I also had to let them know at my work. I phoned work and told the person who answered that I wasn't coming in because Kelly had committed suicide.

Then I phoned Damian, my son-in-law, and when he answered I said to him, "Damian I need your help to tell Fiona gently, that Kelly has died." He was shocked, said he would and that they'd be down shortly. They only lived five minutes up the road.

Next I called Matthew, but he didn't answer; it went to message bank. I hung up and tried again, not wanting to leave a message. By this time I was getting really agitated, so instead of dealing nicely with it, I screamed into the phone, "Pick up the fucking phone, your sister's dead!"

Then I felt really bad. The policeman offered to go and pick them up for me, but I didn't want a police car to be doing that.

I dialed again, and this time Matthew answered. I think that by then I was sobbing. I said that the police would come and get them, but he said they'd get a taxi.

Meanwhile the ambulance men had removed the tube from Kelly's throat, taken the monitoring gear off and were ready to move her to the bedroom. Following me back up the passage, they gently lay her on the bed, on top of her grandmother's patchwork quilt, and covered her with a blanket pulled up to her chin, which hid the vivid bruising on her neck. She looked so peaceful as if she was just asleep. Beautiful, as the marks on her throat were hidden.

Fiona, Matthew and Quill seemed to all arrive together and by then the undertakers were waiting outside to collect Kelly's body, to take to Melbourne for the autopsy. They were very gentle with us, and told us to take our time, not to rush.

Fiona came in first, saw Kelly lying on the bed "asleep" and thought all was OK. She said, "Oh, she's alright then." I say, "No, they just needed somewhere to put her for us."

With that Fiona threw herself at the bed, with her arms around Kelly, crying hysterically and then punching the bed. It was terrible to see and hear. Matthew just looked, standing back leaning against the wall, saying nothing.

We all said our goodbyes, and then it was time to call the undertakers in. They came in with their trolley. I turned away, unable to watch Kelly being put into the black vinyl body bag, and being zipped up. You never expect to see one of your children in an undertaker's body bag.

We all stood on the verandah and watched the undertakers load Kelly into the back of the van, and then take her away, our hearts breaking as she left the house for the last time.

***

As a nurse for over thirty years, I'd dealt with death on a regular basis. I'd been to my eldest brother's funeral after he'd died of a heart attack at age forty-four. I'd been to my father's funeral – no tears shed there – and two years before had buried my mother.

But nothing, no one, can ever prepare you for the death of your child. She may have been twenty, legally an adult, but she was still, and always will be, my baby girl.

The next difficult task was to tell Ross's parents, Peter and Jean. I rang Ross's Uncle Jimmy, and asked him if he would go out to the house to tell them for us, not wanting to tell them over the phone.

The ambulances and police cars had all left by this time and we were on our own. Time now to share our grief, and to share our stories with the family. A story we would be retelling countless times over the next weeks.

THE BOYS IN BLUE

Now it's three in the morning,
Soon the sky will be dawning,
Sadly my mind is muddled
(Actually really quite fuddled)
To the boys in blue
I'll say thanks to you
Never forget your faces
As you went through your paces
Now to thank you I must
(For it's only quite just!)
As I shed many tears
And realise my worst fears
You gave us respect
So very circumspect
I'll think of you often
Even when memories soften
Your care and compassion
Which, in your own fashion
Gave lots of support
Even when you felt fraught
Ross and I seem to find
That we're of a like mind
We say thanks to you
You brave boys in blue!

Christine Howard, 6 August 2000

CHAPTER 7

Tears and Bewilderment

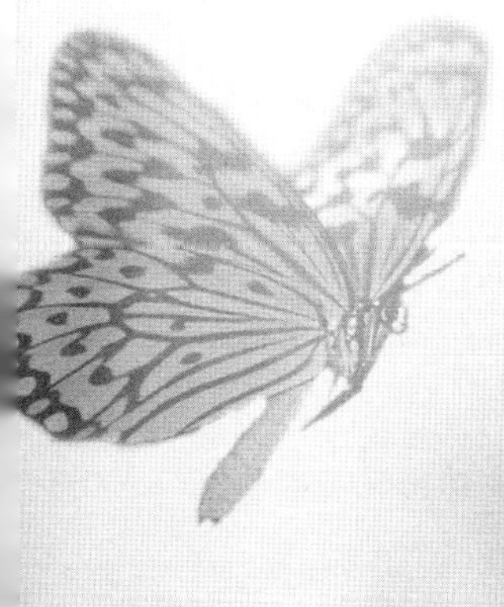

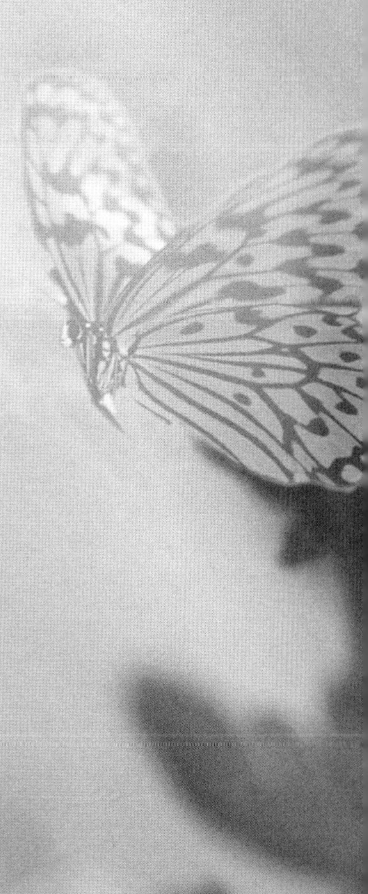

SILVER BED

As I look into the shallow pool of mess.
I stop to think, do they know what's going on?
Or do they need to guess?
Can they hear my screaming yawn?
Do I keep them awake in the early hours of dawn?
I look into the mirror and I see nothing.
There is no change in me, is there supposed to be something?
It won't be long till my life is hanging by a thread.
Till they take my body and rest it on a silver bed.
It's got to stop!
And it will...
It has!!

Kelly Howard, 8 July 1995

CHAPTER 7
Tears and Bewilderment

From the moment we sent Kelly off to the coroner in Melbourne, we were rarely, if ever, alone.

The kettle was kept boiling ready to make countless cups of tea and coffee. The next day Ross's Mum brought in an urn, so there was always hot water for a cuppa, and there were many of these made.

Firstly the close neighbours came to share in our grief, like us, still shaking their heads in disbelief, and to pay their respects. One man said he'd heard Ross yelling from several houses down the street although he didn't think to see what was wrong.

The world seemed surreal, as if I was an actor on a stage, playing some bizarre role. But it didn't end. We sat out on the decking, crying, sharing our story with all that came to offer their condolences.

Ross's parents Peter and Jean arrived, and then a colleague from work came, sent by my boss to bring messages of sympathy from all.

Food started arriving that afternoon, I'm not sure from where, but there was a meal for us that evening, not that any of us really wanted to eat. There was so much, and friends made sure we did eat.

I started making phone calls during the afternoon, calling my brothers and close friends with the sad news. Then it seemed to be appropriate to have a beer or a glass of wine, as we began the futile attempt to drown our sorrows.

We sat around the round table on the decking, all still numb with shock. I'd given up smoking some years before and I was sure that I would start smoking again. However, despite having the desire, the cigarette I tried made me feel sick, so I didn't try any more. It was as if I had a role to play, to look after my husband and children. A few weeks later when things had settled down somewhat, I started smoking again.

Friday nights at our house usually involved an outdoor wood fire, where we unwound from the work of the week over a few drinks. It had become a habit of ours, and there were usually friends who would come to join us. We would sit around the fire, talking and laughing. This Friday night was no exception and only the tears and sombre mood were different.

As the afternoon faded into dusk, Ross, Matthew and Damian set about gathering wood from the woodpile, and building a fire. This time it was with greater purpose than usual – Ross was determined to destroy a particular item.

Years before, my father had made a wooden box, with a lid and castors, which we used as a pantry when we went camping. It was about 18 inches square and stood the same height, with a lift-up lid. It had still been sitting on the decking from our last camping foray.

That morning Kelly had used the box to stand on, in order to loop her rope over the beam of the pergola. It seemed symbolic that she would choose that box over a more stable chair nearby.

Fiona gave the box a big kick, and then others joined in. Between them, they ripped the box apart, stood on it and totally trashed it using their feet and hands, taking their anger and frustration out on it, before it was finally tossed into the fire to burn. It seemed to afford some sense of control in a time of absolute powerlessness.

Then we settled around the fire on our folding chairs, some with rugs to ward off the cool night air. We talked of the events of that day, of how Kelly had been over the past week, how she had appeared to be almost back to her old self again. We talked of the way she had lulled us all into that false sense of security. It seemed that she had come home to say her goodbyes, to leave us with warmer feelings and nice memories. But she had made her decision some time before and knowing nothing of that, we had had no chance to change her mind. Each of us had a story to tell of her in the past few days, but none of us realised what she meant to do.

Once the children were safely tucked up in their beds, we were free to indulge, to swear, sob, scream, as we needed.

Despite having had a Valium sometime that day, I was drinking with no obvious effect (to me). The only sign that I had to tell me I'd had more than enough was my wobbly knees when I stood up to go to bed. My mind was telling me that I should be staggeringly drunk given the amount of alcohol I'd had, yet everything seemed perfectly clear. It was as if the alcohol had had no effect on any of us.

Many more tears were shed, much more alcohol consumed. Gazing into the flames, mesmerised, contemplating our situation and the unbelievable horror of it all.

Then at some point, recognising that I needed to sleep, I said my goodnights to all. Ross opted to join me, leaving the younger couples to watch the fire. I think they stayed there well into to the wee hours of the morning, sharing their grief, and trying to come to terms with the loss.

Alcohol doesn't really drown your sorrows, but for some reason it seems to be the solution of choice. Over the next few weeks we drank much, and burnt up many cartons of cigarettes.

Hugging each other tight in bed, crying together, Ross and I eventually drifted off to sleep. I woke early in the morning thinking it had all been a ghastly nightmare, only to gasp and wail out loud, when I realised it was all too real. I lay there thinking, running through in my head all the events of the day before.

My baby. The beautiful baby girl that I carried in my body for nine months was gone. Never to talk, hug, or laugh with ever again. No more special Kelly birthday cakes. No more cheeky grins or wicked chuckles.

It was impossible to comprehend and understand.

I realised Ross was awake too, and comforting each other again, we cried together and talked until it was time to get up. Life had changed in the worst way imaginable, and it was never going to be the same again.

I don't recall any discussion about Fiona, Damian, Matthew and Quill staying, but along with Joshua and Hayley they all moved back home. I don't know whether it was because they had a need to be with Ross and me, or maybe it was that they felt that we needed the support. It didn't really matter; it was wonderful to have them all here with us.

The little ones, Joshua and Hayley, kept us grounded I suppose, as they needed their routine, although I'm sure they were confused with the constant weeping, and the many visitors.

CHAPTER 8

In Their Own Words: How Others Very Close to Kelly Recall the Final Day

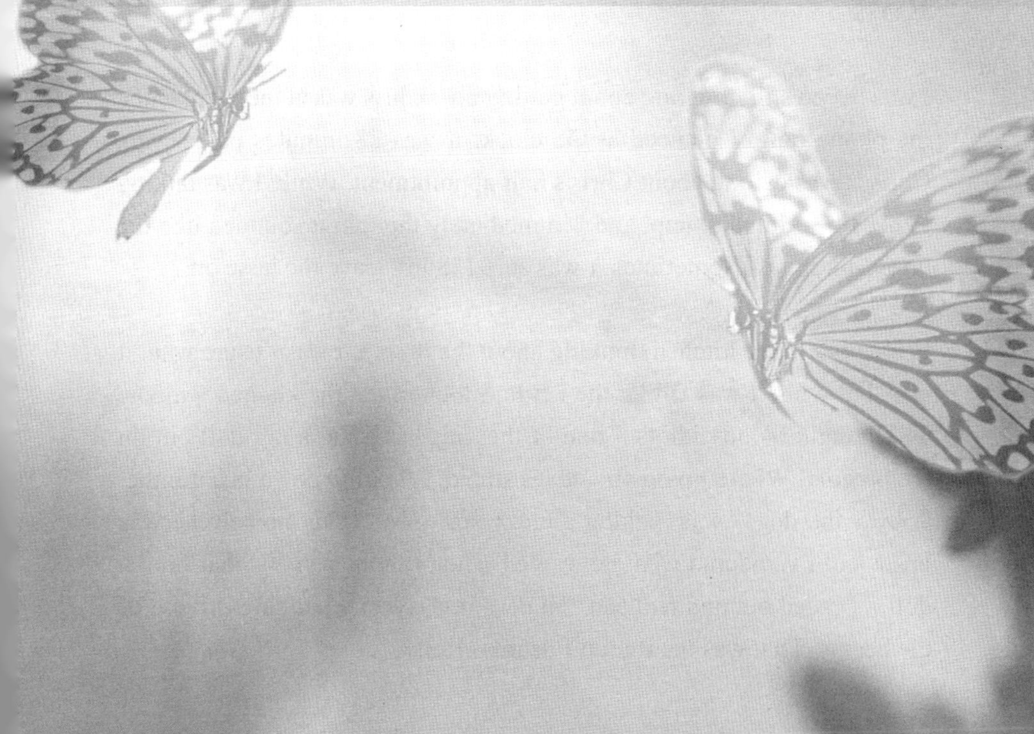

CHAPTER 8
In Their Own Words: How Others Very Close to Kelly Recall the Final Day

Please don't question what I say.
But question how you feel
When you read what I write.

Kelly Howard, 8 July 1997

Ross

I was in bed still, thinking about getting up – Chris was at the gym, when the phone rang. I glanced at the clock; it was 28 minutes past seven. Chris L was calling about Chris's hair appointment. While I was talking to her I heard this thump, and I immediately thought it sounded like the hose shutting off sometimes. I was sure I didn't leave the hose on.

I came out to the kitchen thinking about the thump, I wasn't sure what it was, but while I was filling the kettle, I looked out the kitchen window and thought bloody idiots – one of the kids has hung a rag doll out on the pergola! What's going on – that's stupid, I'll pull it down in a minute. Toby – the dog – was making a crazy sort of a crying noise – he was upset and I wondered what he wanted. Then I thought NO – that's not a doll – I raced out and realised "NO!" – it was Kelly hanging off one of the beams. That was the thump I heard – Kelly …

She'd tied a rope around the beam and she'd used a box that Chris's Dad had made to stand on. Oh shit, oh my God she's hung herself!

I screamed my lungs out, there was nobody around but I wanted help, I yelled, "Jesus, just somebody, bloody hell! Isn't there anybody around?" I'm yelling and yelling – so I lifted her up – I've got no idea now how I did that, not now.

I remember about a week before, we were just talking and she had asked me if I could show her how to tie a nooses knot, and I said, "No! I'm not showing you that!"

She'd used a long bit of rope, tied it at one end, put it over the beam like a loop, put her head in the other end and then jumped off the box.

I screamed and screamed and screamed, there was nobody around! I don't know how I lifted her up and got her down.

I got her on the decking and I said, "Kelly, bloody wake up! Stop it!" And then at the same time I thought, "Bloody hell, she's dead!"

I carried her inside the house, I don't know why I did that and I was thinking about how she'd be embarrassed because her pajama pants were falling down, oh shit, they keep falling down.

Then I rang 000 – no it wasn't 000 – there was a number that used to be on the side of the ambulances and cop cars everywhere – nobody seems to know what it was now, but I rang that number and I got this lady on the phone, she was very nice and I told her what had happened.

I'd calmed down a bit then, and Kelly was lying on the floor. She asked me if I knew how to do CPR, and I said, "What do you mean – oh well OK."

She said, "Check her mouth, has she got any obstruction – can you see her breathing?"

I said, "No – nothing in her mouth and she's not breathing."

She then said, "I'm ringing the ambulance now, start CPR", and she told me how to do it, breathe into her mouth and then press down on her breast plate, and then said, "I want you to keep doing this." Then she said, "Keep doing the breathing, press her chest and keep doing it, you'll hear the ambulance soon, any minute now."

So I kept doing it – I don't know how I was able to do CPR and talk to her, but I managed. She kept talking to me, and then I thought it was starting to work here – I really wanted it to work.

She then said for me to quickly go and open the front door and then continue the CPR until the ambulance men arrived to take over.

So I kept doing it and the next thing I saw two ambulance blokes walking down the passageway. One said "Ross is it?" and I said "Yeah", and he said, "You're the father? We'll just take over now, you just step outside and we will take care of this now."

It wasn't long after that – in fact almost immediately – the cops, detectives were there too, because one of them said, "They're working on her Ross, let's go outside, they'll look after Kelly." So we went outside for a bit and then back into the kitchen and then Chrissie came home.

The morning before this, I had walked out to the kitchen when a voice – Kelly – said, "What are you doing up Dad?" I thought, "Aren't I allowed to be?" So I think it was going to be then, but I surprised her by getting up early. I stopped her.

That night I said to Damian – pointing to the box she'd stood on – "Burn that bloody thing there – smash it up and burn it." Then Fiona and he got into it – we were all kicking it until it broke up and we burned it on the fire we'd made outside.

I'm OK with this now, but if the phone hadn't rung that morning, I'd have been up and she wouldn't have been able to do it. But then she would have done it some other time I guess.

Another thing I remember when we were at the viewing down at the funeral parlour, when I went for a walk in the garden. I felt there was somebody with me and it was Kelly. She walked around the garden with me, she didn't say anything, just held my arm, and then she disappeared. I came back inside and told Chris that I'd just walked around the garden with Kell.

Then one of the guys from the funeral parlor said, "I think it's time we closed the coffin now." I didn't want to do it. A lot of people had been to see her, she looked lovely there, and people kept bringing little gifts to go in the coffin with her.

I remember at the funeral, thinking, "I don't want to bury my daughter." I remember the coffin going down at the cemetery, thinking, "Shit, what am I doing?" It was surreal, there was a nothing feeling again, what was I supposed to be doing, feeling, I didn't know the words to use.

Matthew

More significant to me was the night before Kelly died.

Quill and I had invited Kelly to go to the movies, and then realised that we had double booked when friends arrived. So I rang Kelly and apologised, saying we had to do a raincheck and she was really upbeat, quite OK with us cancelling. She cheerily finished off the conversation saying, "See you later."

On the morning of Kelly's death I remember Mum calling, and hearing her on the answering machine.

Quill and I were living in a studio warehouse, which was one large room with high ceilings, concrete floor and no heating. So we were sleeping in our dome tent, zipped up to keep the heat in.

The phone wasn't far away, with an answering machine. I heard the telephone ring, and then Mum leaving a message yelling, "Pick up the fucking phone, your sister's dead!" She had apparently already called, but we didn't hear the phone.

I remembered thinking, "Which sister?" Both were rather unstable at that time. Quill started crying and got up straight away, she was wandering semi-naked around the room in shock. I sat on the couch calmly putting my clothes on, second-guessing myself, still wondering which sister – I suppose I was in shock too. I think I rang Mum back.

I didn't know what to feel. I remember feeling powerless – knowing my sister was dead – and thinking what was the hurry. Quill was rushing me as well. I don't recall how we got to Mum and Dad's, I suppose we got a taxi. It was all a blur.

When I got to the house, Kelly was still on the floor, they were just getting her ready to move to the bedroom. There seemed to be a lot of people around, mostly in uniforms.

I had nothing to do with moving Kelly – moving from the floor near the laundry doorway to the bedroom. That was happening at the time I got there to the house.

When she was in the room, I remember going in there for a while, resting my hand on her forehead – her cold forehead. She'd been dead a while. That's about it – I don't remember much else.

One policeman offered to make me a cup of tea and I said, "Don't worry about it, I know my way around the kitchen."

After the ambulance men moved Kelly to the bedroom, I went in and spent some time with her, stroking her head and talking quietly.

Much of that morning is a blur; I don't recall Fiona and Damian arriving, or Kelly being taken away.

My memories seem to be all blended in together; we spent so much time at Mum and Dad's house over the next few weeks.

Later, when we were all outside on the decking, someone kicked the box that Pop had made and Kelly had used to stand on, and then Fiona was kicking it. Damian and Dad joined in and the box was destroyed. We burnt the pieces on the fire that evening.

That evening is hard to recall, although I do remember getting drunk. Mum gave me a Valium saying, "This will help you sleep." Quill and I stayed upstairs that night. For me that was pretty much the cement in my relationship with Quill.

A lot of the time after Kelly's death I spent drawing, and drinking beer and coffee. We also went to the Nash (The National Hotel) a lot too in those weeks. I remember writing something to read out at the funeral.

When we were decorating the coffin at the funeral home, Kelly had just come back from the coroner in Melbourne, and they had started getting her ready. Someone came out and said we could go and see Kell.

So we went into this room just off where we were doing the coffin. She was lying on the steel trolley with her deb dress on. Her head was resting on a block of wood and you could see the "Y" incision on her chest – taped up – I felt there were organs missing, it was just cobbled up with big ugly stitches.

Also I could see the large black numbers written on her right thigh – her identification number from the coroner's – through the dress, and it was really upsetting to see my little sister like that.

Fiona

Damian came in and said, "Your Mum's on the phone, your sister's dead!"

I said, "What, wait, what?" Moments before I was lying in bed, contemplating whether to get up, or to sleep in. I asked if I could ring Mum – I don't really know what I did. I know that I got up and tried to go through the door that we had just closed off, and I couldn't get through it. I think the kids were up; yes, Damian was up with them.

Then I dressed, jumped in the car and the windscreen was fogged up, from the night before, or it was raining, or perhaps it was just me crying, as Mum said it was a clear morning – no rain.

I drove down to home, pulled up and saw an ambulance out the front. I got out of the car and I walked inside. I think I walked straight through down the hallway and there were people there, and then I looked into the bedroom and there was a man in there – I think it was an ambulance man with her. Kelly was lying on the bed, and I thought she was all right, she was still alive.

I said, "Oh, she's still OK," and Mum said, "No Bluey, she's not, she's gone." And I thought, "Oh fuck, she's dead!" Then I started crying, and I went over to the bed, and I remember kneeling beside it, pounding the bed with my fists saying, "No Kelly, no, no!"

I was in there for a little bit and there were two people floating around, I don't know if they guided me out or if I walked out on my own.

I came back out to the kitchen; I saw that Dad wasn't OK. And I don't know, there were other people in the kitchen, I remember having a conversation with the two policemen.

One of the detectives had a conversation with me out on the decking about his brother dying and how I should make sure that these guys (Mum and Dad) got counselling – he said we all should get counselling because he took seven years to do it, and he wished he'd done it sooner.

Damian had organised the children; I can't remember when he walked in, and I can't remember Matt coming in. I remember Damian came over. It's all a blur really.

I remember going to get some petrol in the car with Damian, and looking at the clouds and thinking, "Wow"'. It was just so surreal. Not really sure how I should react. I didn't know how I was supposed to feel.

I don't know who picked up the children, but I remember taking Josh up the backyard, sitting him on my knee and explaining to him that Aunty Kelly wasn't here anymore. I sat there with him, and I cried with him. I think he asked a couple of questions, "Why?" and "What does it mean?" and I tried to explain in a nice child-friendly way. He just sat there and let me cry. Then I got up and joined everyone drinking on the decking. I didn't go home and get any clothes, I think Damian went and got clothes for the kids and us.

Damian was working with Howard Gardening, and the night before Dad and Kelly had dropped him off. I was getting the kids ready for a bath, and I had two little kids naked, and they ran out to meet them. So they got to see Kelly the night before she died. They went up to see her, to say hello and then goodbye.

I don't remember what we ate, but I remember people were there, making us eat. We also had to think about doing something for Hayley's birthday the next day.

I also remember driving around to Becky's house that night – she only lived around the corner – to see her and tell her face-to-face. I didn't want to tell her over the phone. I had rung her first to ask if she was at home. She was very helpful and supportive over the next weeks. When I took Josh aside to tell him, I also took myself away for a little while and made some calls to tell friends.

That night, when everyone had gone and it was just the family left, we sat around the table on the decking still drinking. Mum got us all a Temazepam to help us sleep. We let it go a bit long before going to bed and by then we were all going a bit loopy.

I don't remember going to bed, but the morning after was Hayley's birthday. The house was quiet and Josh was the first one up. So I got up and he was riding his little blue and yellow plastic bike around the house, and he was talking. I wondered who he was talking to, but he was definitely having a conversation with someone. Riding around on his little bike chatting away.

So I followed him and he went through the kitchen and then the lounge room, he didn't know I was spying on him. I was hiding so he couldn't see me. He rode up to the stairs, got off his bike and climbed up three steps and then sat down. Then he shuffled across so there was enough room for someone to sit beside him. And then he was talking, and I realised he was talking to Kelly – it was really freaky. But he had a full-on conversation with her.

So then I went into Mum and Dad's bedroom and said, "Are you awake?" Well they were but they weren't. Then I told them all about Josh's conversation with Kell and how freaky it had been.

Despite being in an alcoholic haze, we continued to function over the next days. Getting the photo boards ready, sorting through all the family photos was good.

I remember going into town to buy clothes for the funeral. Decorating the coffin, going into that room at the funeral home with Matt; and us getting really upset when we saw the numbers (that were written on her thigh from the coroner's) through her dress.

Susan

The day started the same as every other day; mug in hand, I opened the front door to drink in the early morning light and peace on the verandah before my gorgeous children rose and the bustle began.

As I glanced across the street my heart lurched. I knew this wasn't going to be any ordinary day. What I saw spelled tragedy. A line of cars parked in front of Chris and Ross's

I'd seen the same line of cars dozens of times when I was the person in blue attending a family tragedy. I didn't know who, but I knew someone had died. A marked police car, unmarked cars that would have held grave-faced suited detectives and a very plain white windowless van. The van was there to transport a body to a funeral parlour.

My heart lurched again as I saw Chris walk up the path to her own front door and quickly disappear inside. What anguish would greet her. Was it Ross or Kelly?

A neighbour crossed the road and sat with me, concern on her face, and asked if I knew what was happening. Another neighbour walked up my front path to enquire if I knew what was going on. All I could say is that I didn't think it was good.

My little kids were awake and while we were saying good morning with cuddles and laughs, the phone rang. I knew before I picked it up, that it was Chris. I remember that call as if it was yesterday; her anguished voice asking me if I could come over because Kelly had hung herself. It had come to this for beautiful Kelly, victim of abuse, tormented and unable to get the help that she needed from the healthcare system. The beautiful portraits I had taken of her just a short time ago flashed before me as I arranged for my neighbour to stay to look after my family.

The front door was open and as I walked in I saw men standing silhouetted against the early sunshine that was pouring through the windows of Chris and Ross's back room. I don't remember their faces as I walked toward them or what they were wearing. I remember the noise of Chris howling from another room and Ross's expression of pure grief and disbelief as he came through the sliding door from the deck.

Time stopped as I stood quietly with my arms around Ross, my thoughts running a million a minute. You can't say, "Are you alright?" because you know it's not all right. You can't say you're sorry because it just isn't big enough. I turned around to see Chris, face ashen and crumbled; her heart breaking before my eyes. Her baby was dead. No cuddle could ever take away the pain.

After a moment Chris told me that Kelly had been found by Ross hanging like a rag doll from the pergola, just under the oak tree. She said that the ambulance men had worked on her to bring her back to life, but it hadn't worked.

I got a chance that morning to say goodbye to an extraordinary young woman, who if only things were different, would be living a happy joyful life now. Instead, she was laid out on one of the single beds, looking like she was pretending to sleep and trying to ignore all the fuss, but with the telltale bruising and swelling across her throat.

I was oblivious to anything else around me and I don't know if anyone else was in the room, other than Kelly. Kelly was slightly warm but with a chill to her skin as I touched her cheek and stroked the back of her hand, willing this not to be real. Her face was so calm and serene and I knew her soul was there and that she had her arms around her parents, trying to give them whatever comfort she could.

Kelly is still around watching her family in the guise of the soft wind, the flutter of butterfly wings and the cooing of white doves. She would be watching over everyone and would most likely have had many a giggle watching Josh and my son Hayden as they learned how to tend over the gardens she'd worked on as the "K" in RCMFK Howard Enterprises.

Kelly would be so very proud of Chris and Ross, and her big brother and sister, Matthew and Fiona, for the way they have managed in the aftermath of her loss. She would be proud of the way they have let her go, but let her live on in their day-to-day lives.

She would be especially proud of her Mum Chris as she embarks on her long dreamt of book. If that book succeeds in helping people understand the warning signs so young lives may live on beyond the blackness and desolation that Kelly went through before she chose to take her own life, Kelly's legacy will live on in the lives of countless families.

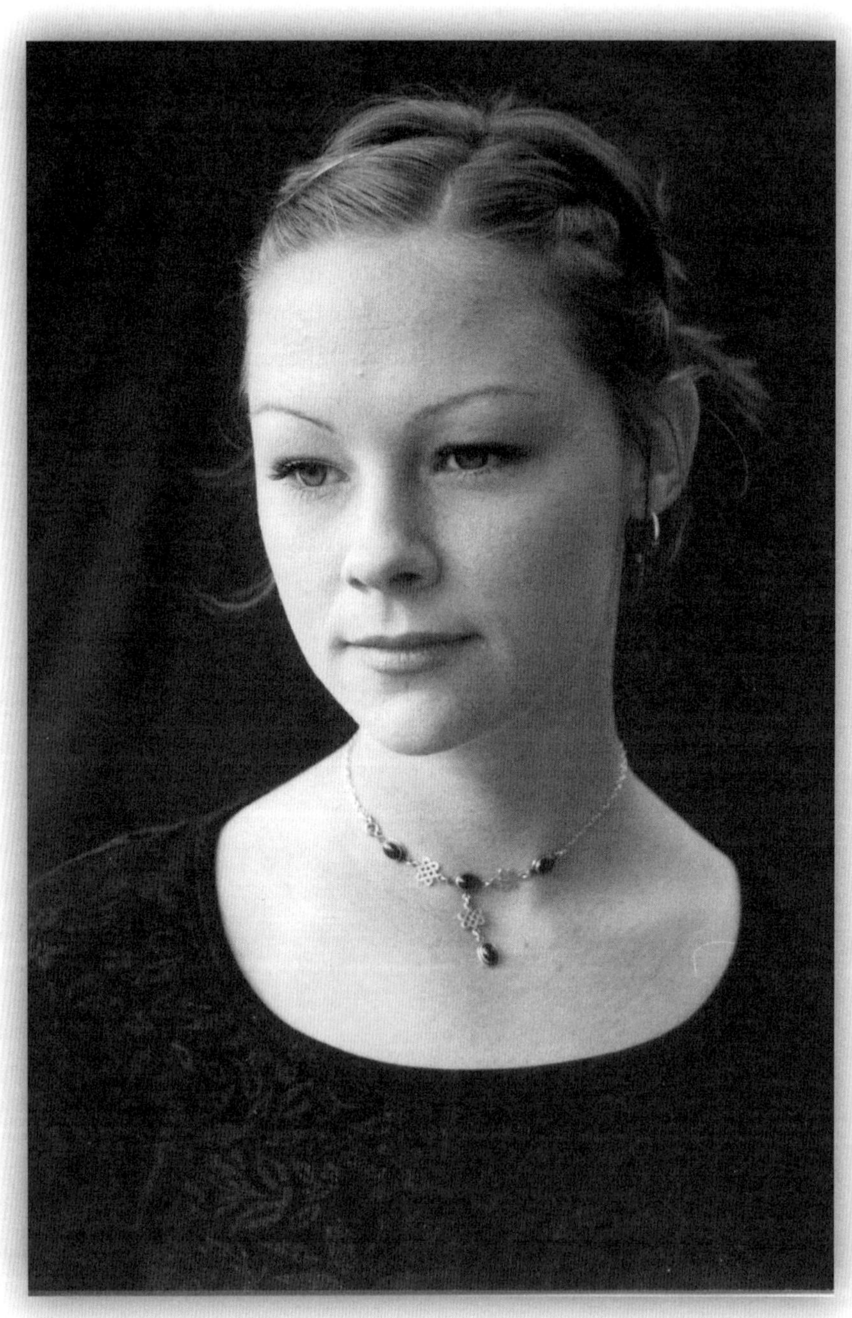

CHAPTER 9

The Morning After

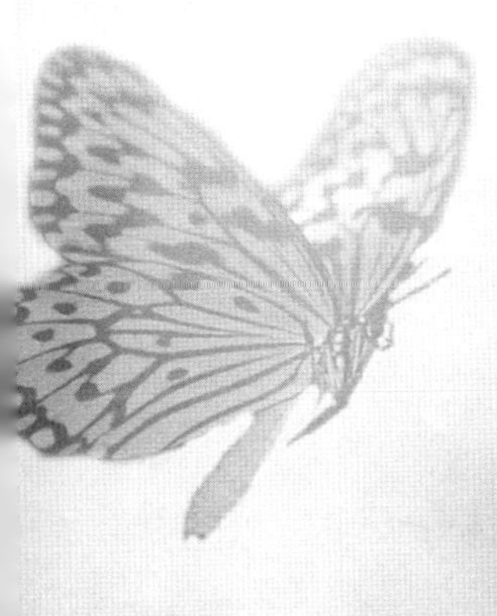

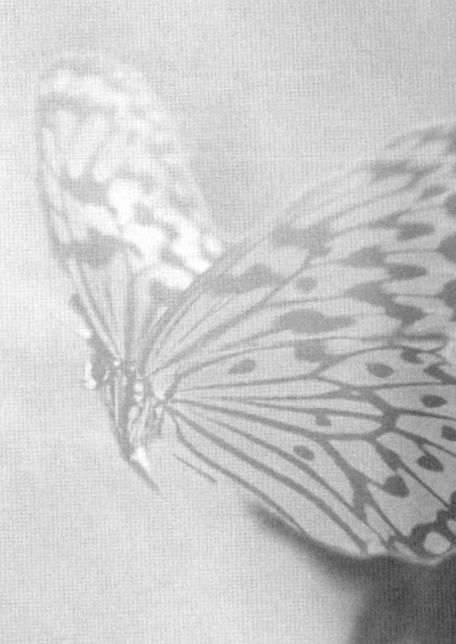

WHEN I DIE

When I die, I don't want people to feel sorry for me,
Just maybe a bit of understanding
I love all my friends, and can't describe the love I feel
for my dear family.
If I die, I'd like to wear my deb dress cause
my favorite Mum made it,
And I love her so much, and my brother,
and my Daddy and my sister.

Kelly

CHAPTER 9
The Morning After

Once up and dressed, I opened the front door to get the morning paper, to find a casserole on the verandah and that someone had laid flowers on the footpath at the front gate. We were being cared for.

My cousin and his wife arrived, the first of numerous visitors that day, bringing a casserole too. Eventually I left the front door open, it seemed more welcoming to the many who came. That set the pattern for the following days, as the doorbell rang frequently with either visitors or a florist with another bouquet of beautiful flowers. After a few days, we ran out of clear spaces to put the flowers, so they were lined up on either side of the passageway to the front door.

We were never alone; there were people – friends and family – there from early morning to late at night. So many cups of tea and coffee, glasses of wine and stubbies of beer consumed. Thankfully we didn't have to think about preparing meals, as there was plenty of food provided for us.

That Saturday was a special one for our family, as it was Hayley's second birthday. Somehow we had to find the strength to be as "normal" as possible for a little girl.

Susan, a dear neighbour, looked after her whilst we got ready for the party. I went over to collect her, and as I was opening our side gate, carrying Hayley back, she put her little hand on my cheek and looked at me saying, "No more kying?" (crying)

I tried really hard not to, for her sake, but it really was impossible.

We had party food and a cake, wore silly hats and danced around to make a little girl and boy happy amidst such devastating sadness. There were other children there too, keeping the illusion of normality – they didn't really understand what had happened, so it must have been very confusing for them.

I think the party helped to ground us, to keep us in reality, and having the children there, needing routine. They went off to day care on weekdays, had their baths and bedtime stories. Meals at regular intervals for the children ensured that most of us adults ate too, something I think we could easily have forgotten to do.

The phone rang a lot with people calling to express their sorrow. People called in to see us, always asking if there was anything they could do for us. Hugs. We had never experienced such love and caring before – some people had difficulty saying anything so they just cried and held us tightly, physically expressing their sorrow, offering some comfort.

One of my nursing colleagues arrived on the doorstep (with a huge jar of delicious homemade melting moments) saying she'd driven around the block a couple of times as she didn't know what to say to me. I said, "There is nothing really to say – you're here and that says a lot anyway."

My faith in humanity was restored in those early days, with the love and support that was shown to us. We were wrapped in a big blanket (metaphorically speaking) of love and caring.

It helped us that others shared our grief, cried and laughed with us. There was laughter, strange as it may seem, but life does go on. Nothing stops. That first morning, I remember feeling outraged that cars were still driving down the street outside. Didn't they know that my world had just ended, and they were going about their business as normal? I felt that if my world had come to a halt, then so should everything else. But that was only for a short while.

Some of Kelly's friends came that first day, and that evening someone found two large pieces of styrofoam sheeting – four foot square – to use as photo boards. Then we got out the family photos, and pulled out all the Kelly ones from over the years.

Then over the next few days, with Fiona directing, the boards were covered with photos, butterflies and captions depicting the life of Kelly. We had them in the foyer of the church for her funeral where people were able to look at them and reminisce. They have been a wonderful memory jogger and talking point over the years.

As Kelly had been taken to the coroner in Melbourne, we were unsure when we would be able to have the funeral, as there was no definite date for her to come home to us.

Then we started the awful process of organising a funeral. Firstly there was a visit from the people who do the funeral, ensuring that we understood the many little things that had to be done. We had to decide where to hold the funeral, who would conduct it, what coffin to choose, what notices to put in the paper and then where she would be buried. Would she have a grave or be cremated? A headstone or a plaque? The list goes on. It was emotionally exhausting working it all out.

Ross's cousin Christopher was a minister so we decided we'd like him to take the service, but he was away on holidays, so we had an anxious wait for our meeting with him, hoping he'd be OK with it. That probably wasn't a bad thing as it gave us some time to think about how we wanted the service to go. There was another friend – Jenny Dunn – an Anglican minister, who we asked to help Christopher with the service. So we had part of it sorted and we just hoped Christopher would agree. Choosing songs, music to play – everyone had ideas on what had been Kelly's favourite songs.

There was never any doubt in my mind what she would wear – her deb dress. It was a dress she absolutely loved, and she had taken to carting it around with her in a black plastic garbage bag.

On one of her visits in the weeks prior to her death, she'd stayed overnight and left the bag at the base of the stairs. As she'd given so many other things away, and knowing how much she loved that dress, I didn't want her to give it away too. So I took it.

I took the bag with the dress and ran across the street to Susan. I asked her to keep it for me, explaining that I didn't think she'd want to lose it. Strangely enough Kelly never mentioned it, I suppose she thought she had given it away or lost it. She gave a lot away in those last weeks, including her bed.

So I collected the dress from Susan, took it to be dry-cleaned and then to the undertakers ready for them to put on her when she came home from the coroner.

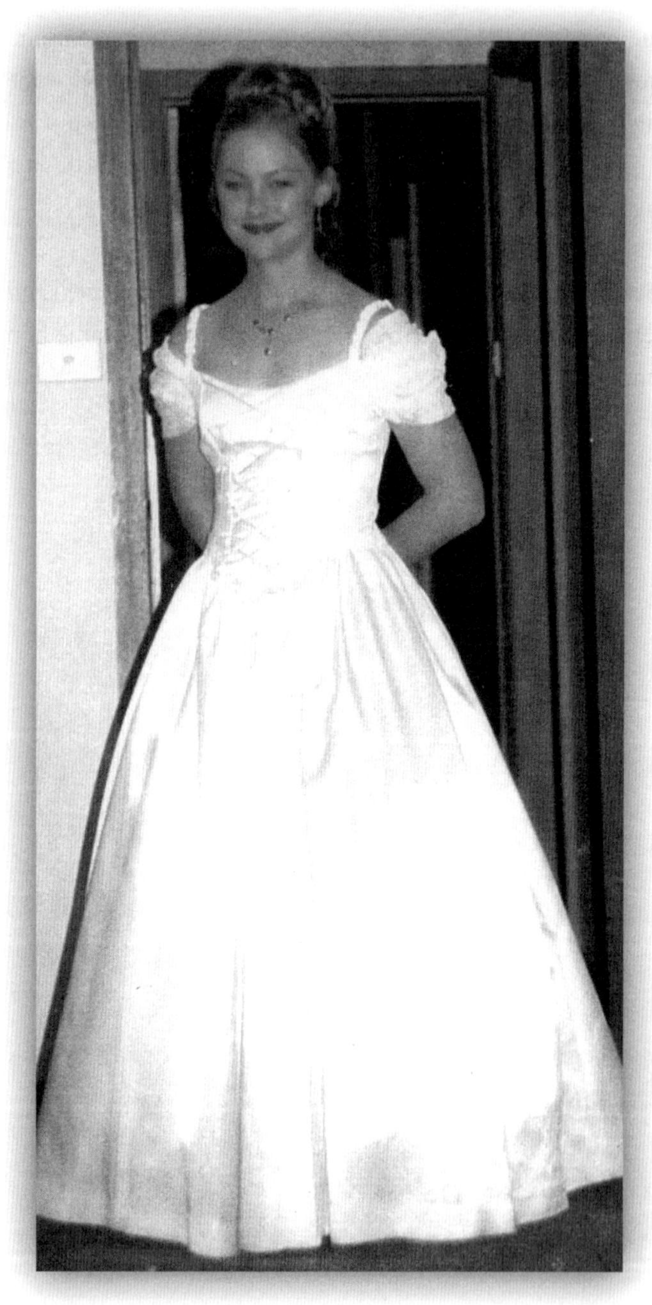

CHAPTER 10

Farewell to Kelly: Our Eulogy

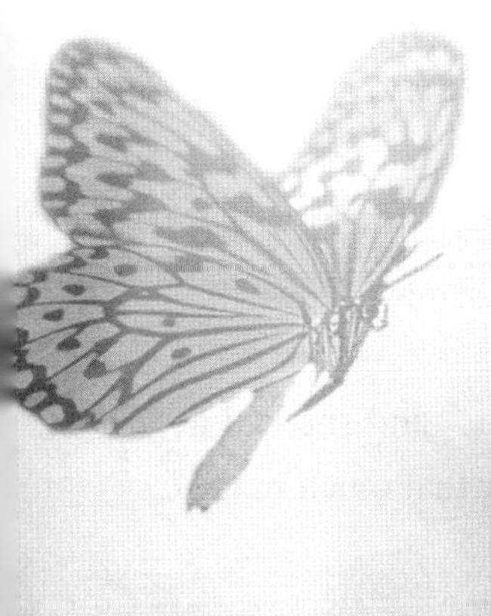

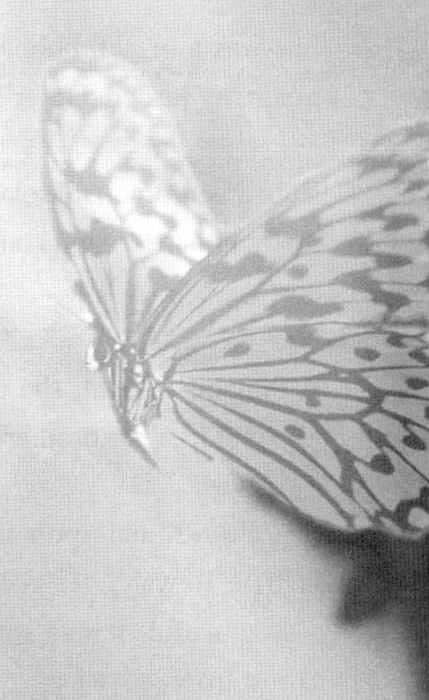

CHAPTER 10
Farewell to Kelly: Our Eulogy

KELLY CHRISTINE HOWARD, 11-11-1979 to 04-08-2000

Kelly was born on Sunday 11th November 1979, just 15 months after Fiona, and one week before Matthew turned three.

There are many adjectives one could use to describe Kelly, but you could probably say that her torment is over, and she is now at peace.

She was a bright, bubbly little girl, with lots of blonde hair – hair that gradually turned darker as she got older, much to her dismay.

Kell was a practical joker – she loved to have a laugh – and she had a really infectious, wicked chuckle. Sadly we didn't hear that much in the past year.

A diligent student, she never gave Ross and I any trouble at school at all – not like her brother and sister!

She enjoyed her sport and loved to compete, from Little Athletics to netball. To watch Kell on the netball court was like watching a ballerina – so graceful. It was something she excelled at and she won best and fairest trophies twice.

A bit of a magpie, she collected lots of pretty things, and jealously guarded her possessions. One of her passions was with elephants; she had quite a large collection of them, in various shapes and sizes. Once she even wrote a letter to the Prime Minister – Bob Hawke – about the plight of the elephants, appealing to him for help.

Her fondest wish was to be an actress. She loved to put on a wig and dress up. She often wore a wig when she went out, especially after she shaved her head!

Rock Eisteddfod was a highlight of her high school years, as well as being involved in other plays.

When Kelly started secondary school, she chose to learn to play the flute. She derived much pleasure, and perhaps some solace from it. We certainly enjoyed listening to her, especially when she played with Fiona and her violin, and on at least one occasion with her cousin Ryan and his saxophone.

Another of her talents was singing, although we never really saw her sing, we have listened to tapes of her singing.

Quite a prolific writer, she kept a journal on and off for some years. It has been quite devastating during these past few days to read some of the entries. She alluded to the fact that she wore many faces, and I believe – sadly – that we never really knew the inner Kelly.

She expressed a lot of her pain through poetry and songwriting, and we have been very proud of her ability with her poems.

Four years ago she performed in what was her greatest role when she made her debut. She was so thrilled with all the excitement and drama associated with it.

She looked beautiful in her dress, a dress she absolutely adored. Those of you who had contact with her in these last few months, will know of her attachment to it, because she carried it around everywhere with her – at least she did until I stole it and hid it from her – and she wanted to wear it a lot.

It must have made her feel special, so she's wearing it today, as she would have wished to. As a mother – and dressmaker – it has been especially gratifying to know that I was able to give her something that she loved so much.

Joshua and Hayley – her nephew and niece – were the light of her life, and she loved to get down on the floor with them, or dress them up and take them out. They thought she was the ant's pants too!

Kelly was a great one for making birthdays special. She made lots of amazing birthday cakes for both children and adults.

Three years ago, Kelly helped Ross start Howard Gardening, and although at times the work was too much for her, she kept trying. There was a time when she didn't contribute, but in the last month when she moved back home again, she started working with Ross and Damian again, and seemed to really enjoy it. She had a feeling for it and always shared her lovely smile with the clients.

We have many memories of Kelly – many of them happy ones – although there are a lot of sad ones too. What we have to endeavour to do now is to try and concentrate on the positives, whilst not really forgetting the negatives. She enriched our lives, and will be sadly missed by many.

Today she is acting in her very own show – and she's got the lead role, as we her family and friends are gathered here to celebrate with her and to applaud her short but eventful life.

She was no angel whilst she was living, but I'd like to think of her as an angel from now on, looking after little ones like she did when she was with us.

She touched so many people with her kindness and sharing.

Thank you.

Chris and Ross

PAIN

Patch my pain through my heart,
When I make a wish, don't tear it apart.
When I look at you
I can see straight through.
I am fearful so do not harm me
I need my happiness can't you see?

Kelly Howard, 20 August 1995

CHAPTER 11

Epilogue

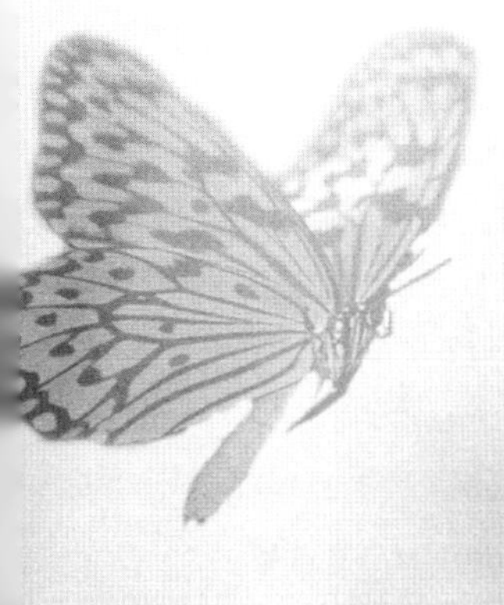

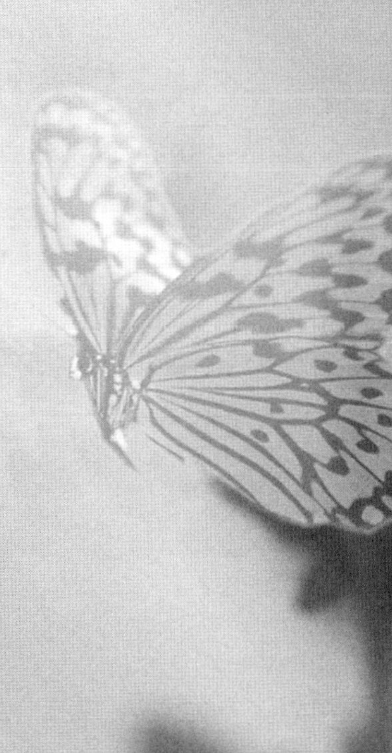

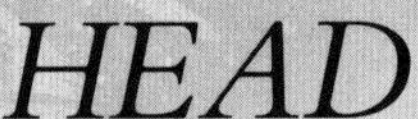

HEAD

I need to take my head off and hang it up.
I want the purity of the cleansed air to free it of all sadness.
It is dark, but when the sun awakes I want it to
Beam its golden rays into my clouded mind.
I now crave for my starving cranium
Which has been stripped of any unhappiness.

Kelly Howard, 17 December 1995

CHAPTER 11
Epilogue

It still feels unreal at times. It's like a bad dream – or a nightmare. But then I wake, and there's reality again.

Starting this book, I've looked back at some of my early journaling and I cringe, thinking of how I or we should have done things differently and then maybe we would still have our Kelly here.

But hindsight is a wonderful thing. We did the best we could, with what we knew at that time, so there is no point in beating ourselves up for what we didn't do. Kelly gave us so many verbal, non-verbal and physical cues that we didn't pick up on.

None of us realised the true state of her mental health or the severity of her illness. Or even that it was an illness. We didn't really think in terms of wellness or illness; people were just classified as "nuts" or "off the planet". Perhaps even an embarrassment. We'd often look the other way.

Whilst mental health is a real concern, not all who die by suicide are mentally ill. Suicide is often seen as a solution to a problem, and when an individual's capacity for coping – with whatever it may be – diminishes, they become exhausted.

According to Mental Health Daily, other causes can include bullying; a traumatic experience such as losing a job or post-traumatic stress;

personality disorders; drug addiction or substance abuse; unemployment; relationship problems; social isolation and loneliness; terminal illness; chronic pain; financial problems and side effects of prescription drugs. *<mentalhealthdaily.com>*

As a family, we accepted that Kelly had been behaving rather oddly for quite some time, but none of us, including the "professionals", really understood that she was ill. She wasn't just behaving badly; her behaviour wasn't something that could be turned off or on. Kelly was suffering and that spilled over into some bizarre behaviour.

She was prescribed medications, antipsychotics I believe, although it's a mystery to me why a doctor would do that when he says there's nothing wrong with her! Apparently Kelly wasn't taking her medication anyway – she was selling it to her friends!

It's difficult watching your child self-destruct in front of you, made even harder when the "professionals", who are there to help, refuse to listen to the family. Surely the ones closest should be believed when they say that this is not normal behaviour. But, because Kelly was an adult, the hospital psychiatrist wasn't interested in what we, her closest family, had to say. It counted for nothing in his eyes because he was the expert, the authority, and he knew what he was doing.

Powerless. We were so powerless.

When it was apparent that Kelly was unwell, and that we were not equipped to handle it, we sought help from those who dealt with this sort of thing, that is, the mentally unbalanced. We expected to find more than we got.

Am I bitter? Perhaps a little, although now, most days, I find I can forgive their ignorance and callousness.

I didn't know what to do, or how to handle Kelly's behaviour, so I started ringing the professionals and saying, "She's doing this now. What should I do?" I called frequently, asking for help, looking for something to make a difference. I felt I was making a nuisance of myself, but I didn't really care. I'm not normally one who demands attention, but instinctively I knew that I needed to make a noise.

It wasn't pretty watching my daughter self-destruct, but I attempted to find solutions, to get help. Looking back, I ask myself if I could have done better. The answer is really unknown; I did the best I could at the time.

It haunts me at times, to think that I hadn't kept up with current trends, and that I was hopelessly outdated in my knowledge of suicide. When I was a very young nurse, we were told that people who talked about taking their life by suicide rarely followed through.

So when Kelly told me she was going to kill herself, I said, "OK dear!" I wonder what it must have felt like to have your mother agree to such a drastic step, and to seemingly not care about the outcome.

So yes, I feel guilty that I didn't do enough to keep my daughter alive. But I'm not totally consumed by it. I will always have that guilt, but I don't let it control who I am.

This book has not been written as simply a sad story. I believe that Kelly's story can make a difference in the lives of others, and that is why I have written it. Kelly loved helping others, and my hope is that this story will be of some help to others.

As a family, we have been blessed with so much love, help and support, and I know that there are people out there who don't have access to such support.

By sharing this story, I hope that it can give comfort to others and, perhaps, even save a life. I may never know, and that doesn't matter. I'd like to think that Kelly's story can make a difference, and that even though she isn't physically with us, she is helping.

There is a lot of information and support available now, and suicide is also talked about more openly but, sadly, there are still too many of our loved ones taking the option of suicide.

Suicide prevention strategies should be taught in secondary schools like first aid. If this was the case, the chances are a lot of us would find ourselves using these tools with people we know. Simply knowing what to say, or what questions to ask would help take away the fears associated with talking about suicide to someone you believe may be at risk.

Our lives are littered with decisions we've made, that when we re-examine them, we see were flawed. We can keep beating ourselves up for not doing this or that, but the reality is we work with what we've got at that time. Some things we have to accept, and then move forward. We can't turn back the clock, and wishing it were possible is a waste of time.

Pink Teddy is still with us, and I'd love to hear the stories he could tell, especially the last night they had together. Selfishly I kept him, when he probably should have gone in the coffin with Kell, but I felt our need was greater.

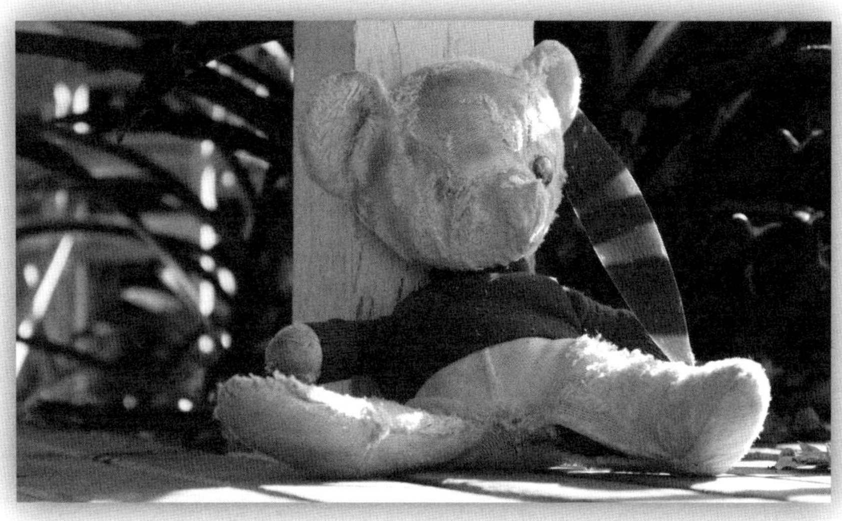

Kelly was born on Remembrance Day, the eleventh day of the eleventh month, so we can never forget her. Often I'll look at the clock and it will read 11.11, and I always say, "Hi Kell". In numerology the number 11 is known as a master number, and the date 11/11 has great spiritual significance.

It has been difficult at times to put this book together, and I've shed many tears as I wrote, and as I re-read. But I sincerely believe that it was meant to be, that I have been obliged to tell the story, and that it will make a difference in this world.

I was blessed to have had Kelly in my life for 20 years; she has taught me so much both in life and in her death. She was our little surprise, but also a gift that gave in so many ways, and keeps on giving – if we choose to accept that.

Thank you for taking the time to read this book, and I hope that you will share it with others.

FREEDOM

Freedom is by choice a destination and
Not something that is hard to obtain.
To survive your unspoken fears is an
Unspoken achievement, to keep them
on the shelf is an act of injustice to
your own self-conscience.
Live happy

Kelly Howard

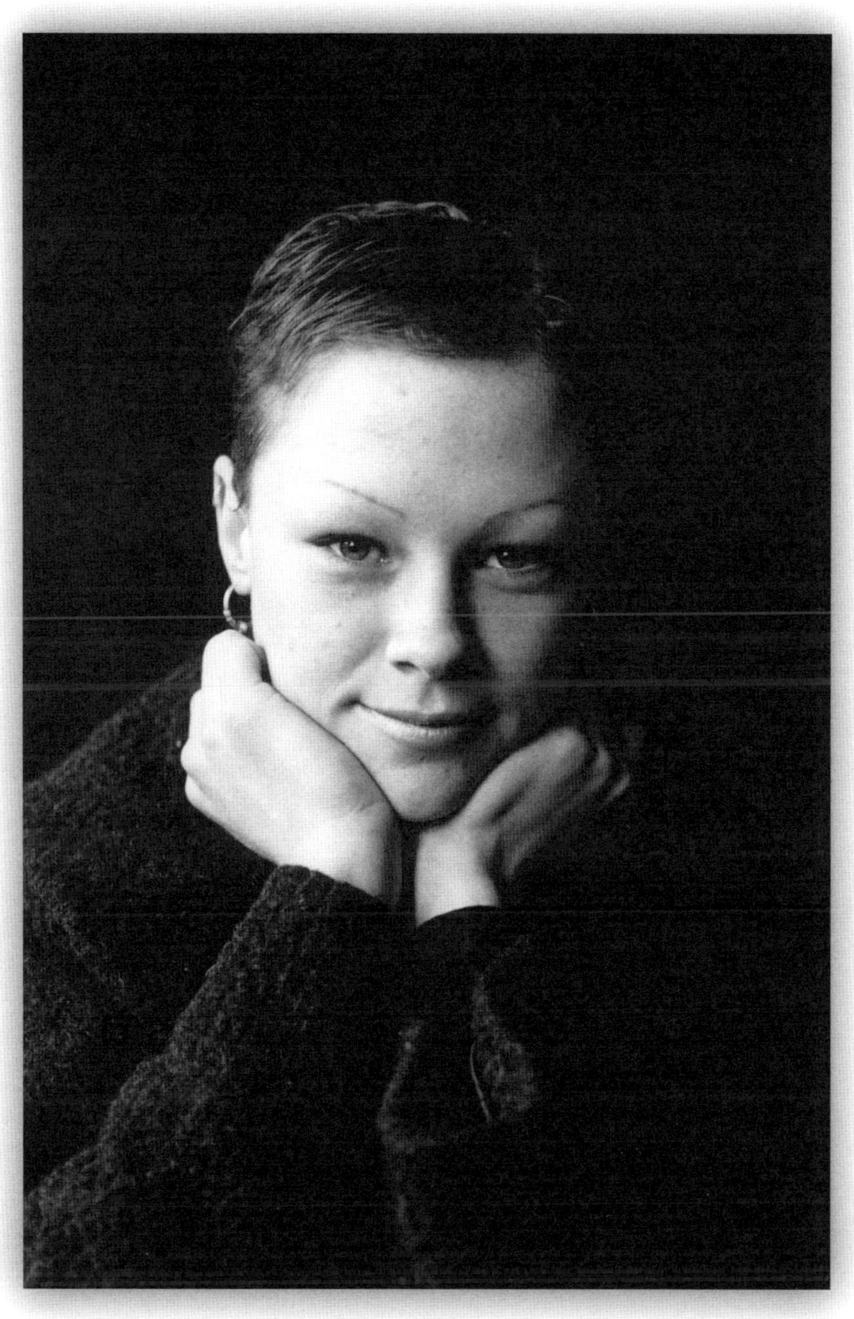

APPENDICES

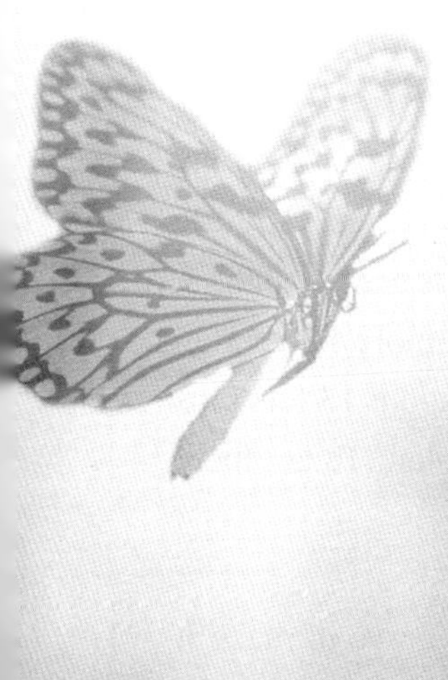

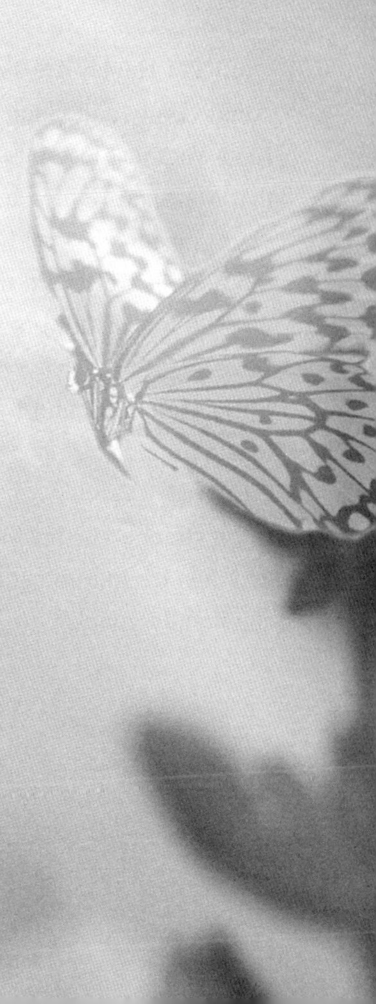

APPENDICES

Appendix (i) Letters to Kell

13th August 2000

Dear Kelly,

Dad, Matt, Josh and I went to visit your grave today.

Quill and Hayley are sick with something like the 'flu. Marnie and Pa, Auntie Betty and Uncle Jimmy came to your grave too. Jenni and little Matt were just leaving – they'd had lunch with you. It was nice to think that Matt had wanted to do that with you. There were more flowers on your grave today – on Friday I'm sure I only counted about 13 lots plus the present we put in the grave so it wouldn't get stolen. Today there were 20 lots of flowers.

Little Matt, Josh and I sprinkled green glitter on your grave to make it look a bit nicer.

It felt strange visiting you there, it doesn't seem real yet, but every now and then it's like someone has punched me in the gut and I think, "Shit, she's really gone!"

We came home and Dad went for a walk, Fiona and Damian have been griping at each other all day. Fiona got out the olives, dip and cheese, so I got out the red wine.

Dad came home and brought out a bottle of champagne – we seem to be trying to make ourselves feel better (it's not really working!)

The doorbell rang and it was Jenni and little Matt with their new dog "Jack" (a Jack Russell terrier). Then Chris L came, so we all had a drink. Damian went out and got fish and chips, Chris went home while Jenni and little Matt stayed.

Earlier today Hannah came, followed later by Simon B, then Wendy and Murray came and stayed for a short while before going home to Kaniva.

It has been rather amazing – quite mind-blowing actually – the amount of love and support we have had since you went. I keep thinking that you would be amazed and surprised if you had had any idea that it would be like this, and that maybe if you had had any inkling, you may not have done it!

Wishful thinking really, I guess I'm just selfish and want you back here with us.

Love Mum xxx

***

20 August 2000

Dear Kelly,

Well another week gone, although in many ways this one has been easier. This afternoon is the first time I've been really alone since you left us. It feels strange – this aloneness – yet I always used to like being alone. While I do not dislike it, it feels odd, like I'm on tenterhooks waiting for something momentous to happen.

Matt and Quill have come home and I feel so sad that you are not here. I feel so much sadness that you have gone for good. I can't seem to stop crying. I think that you would not like me to be crying so much but I can't help it.

I am waiting for Fiona and Damian to come with the kids so I can feel OK. I've rung her several times and she will bring them home soon. I'm really just a wuss.

I love you so much that I can't really express how much.

Love Mum xxx

***

21 August 2000

Dear Kelly,

Well today is Fiona's 22nd birthday – her first without you. I've tried to make it special for her. So far Damian and I have cooked her bacon, eggs and pancakes for breakfast with Joshua helping by serving it to her in bed.

Dad and Damian have just finished packing the back of the work vehicle (they cleaned it out on the weekend), but they still haven't left for work yet and it is nearly 10.30. It has been hard for Dad to get going lately, they started back at work last week, but had rather delayed starts most mornings.

I am starting back at work tomorrow, I took today off because it is Fiona's birthday. I've done a couple of platters of cheeses and salads and we've got champagne, and we are all going to meet up above Eastern Beach to have a picnic lunch. She doesn't know about that yet, and I hope we can get her there and make it a surprise. At least it appears to be a beautiful day – the sun is shining and it is almost warm.

We have decided to clean up the side area off the kitchen. I want to have it paved, and Dad has drawn up some plans. We will get rid of the plum tree and most of the other plants around there, as well as the herb garden. Then we will probably put a water feature in, pave, make some sleeper seats, and have somewhere to plant some of the plants we were given when you died. So it will be almost like a memorial garden for you.

Love Mum xxx

***

5 September 2000

Dear Kelly,

Well it's been quite a while since I sat down and wrote anything. Where do I start?

Today I actually braved the dining room at St Johns for morning tea, sat and had a cuppa with Helen. I feel like I'm on display – "Look, there's Chris – her daughter killed herself you know!" Although they may not be saying anything like that – it could be just my paranoia. Ha ha ha.

I had coffee with one of my reps today, and we talked about you and all that has happened. It's OK to talk about it at the moment, but some days I find it hard to keep the tears at bay.

Yesterday Jenni and little Matt came after work – he's having a hard time coming to terms with your death. Jenni said his doctor had suggested writing things down, and then burning them. So I mentioned that Hannah had given us a pack of joss paper for that purpose, and I gave Matt a handful of papers so he can do just that.

Margaret our counsellor had given us a model of grief and some of the emotions associated with it. We discussed it with Matt and explained to him that it is normal to feel all or some of these emotions at varying times.

Sunday was Fathers' Day, and a very sad one it was for Dad this year. His first without you was very quiet.

Quill, Dad and I went to Fagg's and bought a three-sided garden arch for our front gate, it looks great as it goes over both paths. Quill planted the climbing Masquerade rose, which should look good in a couple of years.

Fiona, Damian and Hayley went home for the afternoon; Josh was asleep on the couch and when he woke up he became hysterical because Fiona wasn't here. I think he thought she wasn't coming back like you didn't. We couldn't console him and had to call Fiona to come and get him.

They all ended up staying at their house; I packed a hamper for them as Fiona had spent all her housekeeping money for here. But it is good they have gone home, I'm not sure if they stayed because Fiona needed us, or if she didn't want to leave us alone. Whatever, we are all managing OK now.

Must go now.

Love you heaps, Mum xxxx

***

17 September 2000

Dear Kelly,

Even though I haven't written for quite a while, it doesn't mean that I'm not thinking about you. You have been occupying my mind pretty much of late, and I guess that will continue for a long, long time yet. Dad doesn't seem to be coping very well at times, but then at others he seems quite OK with it all.

I was concerned that Fiona and Matt hadn't done anything about getting counselling, but when Dad and I saw Margaret on Tuesday, she told me not to nag them, and that maybe they are getting enough counselling from us at the moment. So I guess I have to go along with that for now. Quill was going to see someone last week, but I forgot to ask her how she went.

This weekend has been particularly hard for us, as on Friday night it was the opening ceremony for the Olympics. Dad and I couldn't help but think all the way through it that you would have loved it. But I guess you will have seen it anyway – if you can see from where you are?

He was rather grumpy this morning, as I had decided to go to the gym for a pump class and maybe go for a coffee with Helen and Merri afterwards. Helen wasn't there so Merri and I went for a coffee and chat. I filled her in on all that has happened over the past six weeks since your death.

She spoke of her admiration for me – and the family – for the way we made ourselves available for you kids and your friends. I don't see it as something admirable, but rather as the norm – parents should be available and make their homes a "home-away-from-home" for their children's friends.

Becky came over to visit yesterday, and stayed for quite a while. We talked lots, and I showed her some of the writing I'd done when you were going through your really chaotic patch, and she was shocked to read that you'd eaten meat – she rang her Mum to tell her.

Well, tea is ready now, so better say goodbye for now.

Love you heaps, Mum xxxxx

***

19 September 2000

Dear Kelly,

Just a bit of time up my sleeve before tea, so I'm taking the time to put a few words together.

I'm feeling really inspired at the prospect of writing my "book" – you know I've joked for years about doing it, and now I think I really have to. I need to tell your story, and maybe I can help some other Mum who is facing the same sort of personal trauma that I have. You never know, and anyway I feel the need to write – but maybe no-one will be interested in publishing it!

Dad had a bad day yesterday – at least a "down" day – but I guess that is allowed still. I haven't had one for a while, I hope I can keep going as I am, but I seriously doubt it. I seem to be coping reasonably well, but I'm wondering if that is because I'm a mother, and mothers tend to have to cope with lots of horrible shit.

Or maybe it's because I had (subconsciously) thought that I would lose one of my children one day, because of all that shit! Maybe it's like the deb dress – I hid it from you when I found it in the black garbage bag on one of your trips home with lots of bags. I kept it because I knew how special it was to you, and somehow I think I knew I would bury you in that dress.

Mind you – I was feeling guilty a few weeks ago for hiding that dress – I felt that perhaps I shouldn't have because it obviously meant so much to you, and I shouldn't have deprived you of it. But then I thought about how I would have felt if I hadn't been able to find it after you died, and had not been able to bury you in it. That would have hurt so much more, so I'm glad really, that I did what I did.

You looked absolutely beautiful in it in your coffin – a real sleeping beauty with the flowers in your hair, and around your neck, the glitter glistening on your face. Your make-up and hair were perfect – thanks to Fiona who oversaw all that to ensure your final day was just right.

Backing up a bit – I had thought on occasion that I would lose one of you in some way – over the past few years. I suppose it doesn't take Einstein to work that one out – given that Fiona tried to commit suicide, and then you'd tried it too. However, like most Mums – I tried not to be too negative, and hoped that it would never happen. You know that suicide happens, but it is really just a sad statistic until it happens to your family.

Now for some exciting news – Matt got the commission to do the mural at the Nash – at his price. We are really excited for him, coming so close on the heels of the mural at the Belmont Library; it is really great for him.

By the way, Dad visited the Railway Hotel after work this evening as someone had told him that there was a photo of you on the wall there. He introduced himself to the owner and asked about you. The owner asked if he was your Dad, and said that yes, there was a photo there of you singing.

I'm so sorry we didn't believe you – but then you weren't really very believable at that time, and you never really let us know in enough time for us to go and see you performing there. I guess that this will go down as one of my biggest regrets – not ever seeing you sing.

Well I could probably keep writing all night, but I won't, as I need to rest a bit. There is so much more I want to say to you, but I will get to it eventually.

So, good night, lots of love Mum xxxxx

***

2 October 2000

Dear Kelly,

Well time is really flying – it's now eight weeks since you went, and it still seems like yesterday. The past week and a half have been quite difficult at times for me, but that is the norm for Dad. So now I guess I really know how he feels most of the time. It's not good – it means I'm not very productive either at work or at home, and I find that rather frustrating, as I'm sure you know.

Fiona says she is not allowed to grieve – no one will let her talk about you.

Fiona and I tackled your room last weekend, and it was an interesting experience. We sorted through all your things, packed a lot away and put all your clothes out to be washed. It took a long while as we kept stopping to show each other little things. We cried a lot, but we got it done.

Then we washed your clothes. When they were dry, we sorted through them and put some out for the op shop, some we thought Hayley might like when she is older so we packed them away, and others were too full of memories of you for us to get rid of. So we have packed them away nicely in the old suitcases, ready to be tackled some other year in the future, when we perhaps are feeling less raw.

Joshua had his birthday party at home. Damian made and decorated the cake – a pink dinosaur. Josh was very pleased with it. There were lots of kids there for Josh, and lots of presents. It was a good day, but so lacking because you weren't there.

Time has gotten away from me again, must close now. Will write more soon and tell you about "the baby"!

Love Mum xxxxx

***

3 October 2000

Dear Kelly,

I know it's close to the last letter, but I needed to write down what happened today before I forget the little things – as I'm sure I have before.

I had a productive day at work today – got lots done. The cleaner was talking to me about you – asking how I was coping. She commented about me being too young to be thinking of headstones. I said that no one ever really believes that they will outlive their children.

I had several periods where I felt quite low today; however, I went down to my car at lunchtime and wrote in my journal about my feelings. Wrote five pages in all – wow!

Whilst there Matt sent me a message saying, "I love you, Mum," so I replied likewise, and then I rang him anyway.

I am blessed with my children – even you – when you were alive. I know I am biased, but I'm very proud of my children. It's not easy to rise above a background of abuse, but Fiona and Matthew have done, although sadly you were unable to.

Still, the lives you touched whilst you were here on earth are probably countless. Enough to know that when we watch the video of your funeral there are faces there that none of us know, and if all the cards, flowers and letters we as a family received after you died are anything to go on, then you did make a difference to many people.

You meant so much to all of us, and perhaps it is the old story that we didn't really let you know enough whilst you were alive, but talk lots and think much now that you have gone.

I had a counselling session with Margaret after work tonight. Dad was meant to be there too, but he was late home from work. Anyway it was probably better I went alone, as I talked lots, and feel much more at ease tonight than I did yesterday. Margaret suggested that I should write a book – and I said I was.

I certainly feel I need to do something about your death, not to just let it go and try to become accustomed to it.

I have this burning need to make sure that your life was not for nothing, and that you didn't die in vain. I hope sincerely that I can do something to follow on from your death, not to capitalise on it, but rather to make your life – and your dying – worthwhile.

I believe that you did help many people, and maybe made a difference in to their lives. Your friend Emily used you in one of her school projects and gave us a copy.

Even though we never really knew him, except briefly as your boyfriend, Michael has gone on to get a job and to try to make something out of his life for your sake.

The big news now is that Matt and Quill are expecting a baby, and I believe that this baby has been sent to us all for a purpose – maybe to take the harshness away from our grief, not to make us forget or replace you, but rather to give us a new focus, with the advent of a new life.

As Margaret said tonight, this baby will learn to know and love you too, because we will never ever forget you Kell, you will live on in our hearts and memories forever.

Well it's getting late and I should go to bed, as I want to go to the gym in the morning. Dad told me this morning that every morning when I go to the gym he dozes off after I've gone, and then wakes with a fright, thinking he has to go and get you down from the pergola again.

I said I couldn't stop going to the gym, and he agreed, but said that he would start getting up when I do from now on.

The pain goes on and on.

Goodnight, love Mum xxxx

***

8 October 2000

Dear Kell,

Just in time to write a quick letter whilst I eat my breakfast. Then I've got to get ready to go to Chadstone with Kathy, Lauren and Fiona to go shopping.

They were here for a barbecue on Friday night, and Kathy mentioned it. I'm very much afraid I sort of invited myself along, but she didn't seem to mind – well not that I noticed (I wasn't exactly sober you know!) It was the nine-week anniversary of your death, so we put my current favorite CD on – *My Best Friend's Wedding*, which makes me go to mush. So I'd cried a bit too.

Last night we went to the RSL club for dinner, as it was Aunty Robyn's birthday. It was a pleasant enough evening, although Dad had to go outside for a weep.

It is rather unnerving going out to social events now, as you never know when "it" is going to hit you and make you want to weep. It's different at home, in our own environment and it doesn't matter if we cry. But when you are out and feel it coming on and you just can't stop it, it is rather difficult. Fortunately we don't both do it at the same time – now that would be embarrassing for everyone!

Well I had better stop and get ready – thought this would only be a short letter, and I've written heaps already.

Love Mum xxxx

***

9 October 2000

Dear Kell,

Well once again I have some time to write some more. Yesterday was the shopping trip to Chadstone. It was quite relaxing and very enjoyable – we may end up doing it again some day.

Dad went to Marnie and Pa's for lunch and stayed most of the day.

When we got home, Kathy came in for a cuppa; Fiona went home to the kids, as it was nearly 6 pm. After Kathy and Lauren left, I hung everything up carefully on the door outside the laundry.

I went and sat down to read my book, and I realised that I had hung them there to show you when you got home!

That brought the tears again, it just seems so unfair that you have gone and I can never share my shopping with you ever again. I sobbed on Dad's shoulder for a while, feeling so sorry for me – you – all of us I guess.

I don't think I told you all about Joshua on his birthday. I took one of the books you'd left upstairs and wrote in it – "To Joshua love from Kelly," plus I used the card with the number 5 and the superman badge I found upstairs too. When I gave it to him I told him it was from Aunty Kell.

After everyone had left his party, Fiona, Becky, Joshua, Dad and I went to visit your grave and put more flowers there. Once there I nudged Josh and said "Don't forget to thank Kell for the present!"

He stood on your grave, looked up to the sky and bellowed, "Thanks for the present Kell." It was so lovely, then he proceeded to yell out to you about all his other presents too, I had to walk away, it was so touchingly innocent. Becky asked him if you were a cloud and he looked disgusted and said, "No, she's just there – she's everywhere!" So he seems to have it all under control, much better than us adults.

We were never prepared for death as children, not like some other cultures, which I think is very wrong. We don't seem to let our children participate in the grieving process, so consequently as adults we find it uncomfortable to talk to the dead, when in fact there probably really isn't anything wrong with it at all. At least the children associated with this family will find it easier to deal with as adults, I think – or at least I hope so.

Josh asked Becky on Friday night if she missed you, because he does. He said he wished you were here.

The Saturday before last Dad answered the phone to your old boyfriend Troy, who was quite distressed as he had just found a couple of bags of your clothes and a letter to Fiona and Damian in the boot of his car. We told him Fiona was in Melbourne for the day and gave him her phone number. Unfortunately her phone was playing up and she never received any of his calls.

We had a couple from him. Ross felt that he wasn't coping very well with your death, I suppose because he really doesn't have anyone to talk to about you either.

He delivered the clothes to Fiona a few days later, stayed and talked for a while, then left promising to came back and talk some more.

We still haven't had many visits from your friends yet; I think they are scared to come here. "A" doesn't want to come on her own, she's asked Beck to come with her, which she will. Claire still hasn't come in, although I've talked to her on the phone, and seen her, I don't think she's coping very well either.

"L" is obviously not keen on seeing us, as she took a long time to bring your things around, and even then that was only after we'd rung her and asked for them. We called and her flatmate said she was in bed with the 'flu. She then said she'd bring them around, and when she did there was no-one around so she threw them over the side gate, and of course Toby got to them and chewed the arse out of a pair of your shorts! So I wasn't very impressed about that, especially as seeing the bag there reminded me of you and the way you were in those chaotic times, and I got a bit of a fright before I was able to tell myself that it couldn't have been you.

I know it was silly really, but I felt hurt that someone who purported to be your good friend has not even had the decency to call and see if we got the goods OK. Sad.

Well I better go and fold that mountain of washing.

Catch you later, lots of love Mum xxxx

***

15 October 2000

Dear Kell,

Feeling nice and relaxed here at Bellbrae, although a little sad that you never got to see it. Dad and I have just been reading, walking and swimming. It's so peaceful and relaxing.

Your death still hurts, but there is a growing calmness, or perhaps acceptance of the loss. It is something I have to learn to live with, and I suppose it's only natural that it gets easier with time. Although every now and then a memory creeps in, of that day you died, and hell, it hurts so much.

I can look back and recall with absolute clarity certain parts of that day, but other parts take on a surreal or unreal aspect that is not easily remembered. We continued to function – automatically I guess, because that's what we do as human beings. The reality was that all we wanted to do was to turn back the clock and have a second chance with you.

Last night, during the night I was filled with doubts about my ability to actually write a book, but now I don't see why I couldn't. I don't quite know what format my book will take (that's positive isn't it?), and I don't know who will want to read it – other than family and friends. Do I write with changed names, or do I write it like a family biography? These types of questions are endless, and only serve to make me feel unsure again.

I'll say goodbye now,

Lots of love Mum xxxx

***

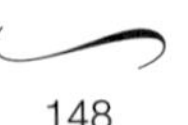

6 November 2000

Dear Kell,

Quite a lot has been happening here in the last two weeks, we've been out and about rather a lot for us.

Last Sunday we went back to the Western Heights Uniting Church for a special service celebrating All Saints Day – which is really on the 1st November. Christopher Howard had invited all families of those who had been buried from that church this year. Marnie and Pa came too. The church was packed.

It was an emotional service, quite lovely, but also very difficult. I could see your coffin there so clearly, and it hurt so much to bring it all back again, just like it was yesterday. I cried for most of the service. At one point we were invited to go up and light a candle for you, so Dad and I went up, he lit a candle and placed it in the sandbox whilst I held his hand and cried.

Really it was good, and it needed to be done – to go back and face the place where you were when we began our final goodbyes. (I'm having trouble seeing the computer screen now just thinking about it!) Dad said he looked to the ceiling in the church and he saw you there, reassuring him that all was OK.

Christopher said he hoped that Dad and I would look on that church as our spiritual home, and I think it will be, simply because we buried you from there.

After church we went for coffee, and then to a home décor place to get some items to make a memorial garden for you. We've planted the rose that Liz gave us called "Loving Memory" and the gardenia that Claire gave us beside the pond at the end of the shed. That way we will be able to enjoy the flowers when they bloom from the decking. We've still got two more plants to go in the front garden; ones that Claire and Audrey gave us.

Fiona was telling us about a dream she had where you came to her to reassure her too. She felt it was so real, and I think she feels much calmer about your death now because of your visit. But maybe I'm being fanciful. Matthew also had a dream that involved you and Pop Nitchie so it is happening all around me.

I am just having trouble thinking about next Saturday – your 21st birthday. It makes me cry every time I think of it, and I feel so sad that you didn't live to see your 21st.

It has become such a symbolic age in our society, that we make such a big deal about it. Fiona and Becky are planning your party – we do intend to have one, even though your physical body will not be here. The plan so far is to go out to the cemetery and light candles at your grave and put lots of flowers on it. A sort of a vigil, but then we will come back here for the party.

It's going to be very hard to cope with this week, especially on Saturday – I bought an extra box of tissues last night, as I think we are going to need them!

Must go now; talk soon, lots of love Mum xxxx

***

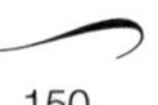

9 November 2000

Dear Kell,

Well your birthday day is getting closer!

I have coped much better than I thought I would earlier in the week – so far. Today I'm waiting for a couple of the girls from work to pick me up and take me to the new clinic at the Mercy Private hospital. Should be interesting.

On Monday I wrote my first decent poem since my thank you to the "Boys in Blue" that incidentally I have never given them. I have called this one "Coming of Age" but perhaps I should have called it "Despair".

It has inspired me to think about writing more poetry, as it is a great way to express my feelings, and to perhaps reach other people.

I will also endeavor to get your poetry published, so it can inspire many people – not just the family. I feel it will be worth it, and that people will really want to read it.

We are gearing up for your party on Saturday evening, although the place here is such a mess. I should really be cleaning it up right now instead of writing this, but it will keep. Dad will have to help me later as it is not all my mess!

So many objects seem to have taken on new significance since you died we relate them to times with you, or occasions. I suppose that is a normal experience with the death of a loved one, but I just hope we aren't becoming obsessive or even pathetic. I don't believe that, but a tiny part of me is asking the question, so I have to raise the issue.

Enough of that now, I really must go and do some work,

Will write more later, lots of love Mum xxxx

COMING OF AGE

These words bring a shiver
And my lip starts to quiver
I've tried hard not to think
Kept pulling back from the brink
OF DESPAIR

Your coming of age
Makes me feel I could rage
The regrets I have felt
Make my soul start to melt
In despair

Those plans that we made
For the hordes to invade
We were all hale and hearty
At the thought of your party
Now despair

Now I keep stopping and sighing
Can't seem to stop crying
Thoughts of the child that I made
Memories never ever to fade
From despair

When you made your decision
With all youthful derision
What did you really think?
When you were on the brink
Of despair

It has been so unkind
To those left behind
To those who have loved you
With never a thought to –
Despair

For yes, we all loved you
And wanted to help you to
Recover from depression
Regain your life's passion
Not despair!

We can't turn back the tide
Nor revert suicide
But still we are yearning
Even as we are learning
Despair

***

19 November 2000

Dear Kelly,

Well it's been quite a while again since I last wrote. I didn't realise just how anxious I was about your birthday until it was over, and I was relaxed again. Everything seemed to take on overly large proportions, as I was so tense.

Last Saturday was Remembrance Day – your 21st birthday.

A day we will never forget. A very sad day for all of us – we were robbed! We were looking forward to celebrating it with you, but that was not to be. So we decided to celebrate it without you anyway. Fiona and Becky did nearly all the organising, invited all your old mates and most of them came. Preparing food and making up salad platters; I couldn't help but think how well you used to make them for me. It was lovely when we worked in the kitchen together – I miss that now.

Claire called in on her way to her Dad's birthday party. Then the others arrived. Once most were here, we all piled into cars and drove over to the cemetery. Others met us there.

We put lots of flowers on your grave, candles, two metallic sprays of "21st" plus balloons. Fiona got one that said "Happy 21st". Becky had one with bears on it and "Be your best friend forever" and I had a heart-shaped one with "Miss you" on it. We couldn't light the candles because it was too windy. We put 21st glitter sprinkles, red lip-shaped and red heart-shaped sprinkles all over your grave. Josh made the ultimate sacrifice and put the last of his dinosaur sprinkles on too.

It was a really sad moment, I felt we shouldn't have to be there and I cried. Most of the others cried too. At one stage I spotted Fiona leaning on the car on her own, so I went over to her, put my arms around her and said, "Don't you ever do this to me!" She replied that she wouldn't and that I wasn't to either!

We came back home and really started to party. More came, some had just missed us at the cemetery. Kristy gave me a green Beanie Bear key ring with "Kelly" on it. Troy came after he'd been to the cemetery and he was terribly upset.

Mel from work came, and Josh went up to her and said, "You know its Kelly's birthday today." Mel said she did, and then he said, "She's dead you know!" – very matter of fact. He was quite excited to be celebrating your birthday, even though you weren't here. Fiona made a butterfly cake and we had to sing happy birthday for Joshua's benefit, but it all seemed right. He handed around pieces of cake, and loaded a plate with about four pieces for himself!

It really was a great party, not just because everybody was having a good time socialising.

We lit candles and had them set all around the decking and some in the garden. The weather wasn't too bad; at least it didn't rain.

There were groups of your friends sitting around telling Kelly stories. They talked about their recollections of you in the months leading up to your death. For me it was lovely to hear them, and to have them talking about you – it would have been healing. I think most of them found it difficult to cope after the funeral, probably because they had not had the experience of losing a close friend.

None of them stayed then, but when they came for your party, they were really having their own version of a wake. It would have really been good for them. Carolyn left three times – she kept coming back!

There were lots of tears and much laughter, and of course lots of toasts to you.

All in all, I believe it was a very good night, just that you weren't there to celebrate with us.

Well, enough for this time – back soon. Lots of love Mum xxxxx

***

26 November 2000

Dear Kelly,

Another week gone and so much has happened. Mostly work related, so I won't bore you with that, except to say that I clocked up 28 hours overtime last fortnight. Don't think I can keep that up for much longer.

I had another session with Margaret. I really enjoy those sessions as I get so much out of them.

Dad said that Becky and Fiona were off to Melbourne to see Tess and Hannah. The girls seem to be helping each other cope with their grief. It is good that they can get together and talk like they do. I just wish that you were really there with them again.

Yesterday I went out to Belmont to order more photos for Marnie, from the ones Susan took. I guess really I've been reluctant to let the negatives out of my sight, feeling that if anything happens to them I've got nothing. Which is actually untrue, but it is the feeling I have – silly or not.

When I handed them to the lady in the shop – even though I knew it was a silly thing to say – I said, "Please take good care of these, they are very precious to me, because they are of my daughter who died recently."

She promised me that she would take good care of them. I left the shop in tears, but couldn't help myself.

On the way home there were highway collectors at the major intersections, and they were collecting for teenage suicide prevention! I couldn't help thinking – I've just given $6000 towards teen suicide – paying for my daughter's funeral!

Afterwards I went to the gym, which has been difficult to do lately, because Dad was so anxious when I left early.

Quill had her 20-week ultrasound scan this week. She and Matt invited Catriona and me too. We were all very excited watching the baby, it looks rather cute with a little pointed chin, which Quill is convinced is like yours Kell. I shed another tear or two at that observation, something I seem to do very easily now.

At last we have something to be excited about, some joy in our lives again.

Must go, love Mum xxxx

***

21 December 2000

Dear Kell,

My letters seem to be getting further apart; maybe I'm adjusting better to your death. I'm still feeling pretty exhausted, it seems to be the norm lately, especially with the hours I've been putting in at work and the quantity of work I had to fit in whilst I'm there, so not surprising.

Feeling very vulnerable now – a combination of being very tired from work and missing you so much at this time of the year. Everything we do now reminds us of you – especially the things we did together last year and how happy you appeared to be then. That was before the rot set in, and you changed so completely from my lovely Kell, my best friend and mate to the stranger you became.

I kept saying, "I just want my Kelly back – the one I used to have last Christmas," and then you died. Now we are left to try and get on with our lives as best we can, and I think we have been managing to do that reasonably well, although not so much these past couple of weeks.

The Christmas cards keep arriving – some with messages of encouragement from friends, and others with good wishes to all of the family including you – from those that don't know you've died. To those we've sent cards back with a note in telling what each member of the family is doing, and including your suicide so that they will know. I did let as many people know as possible, but obviously I missed quite a lot.

Fiona is very unhappy with her life right now; I think it's mainly because she is missing you too. She said last night that Josh asked to go and visit your grave this week, as he hadn't seen you for a while. He has been very good, and next year is going to school. I wish you could be here to see him off, I suppose I will cry when he goes – my baby is really growing up when he goes to school!

Both he and Hayley are getting very tall, it would be easy to mistake Hayley for a three year old as she talks so well and looks older than she is. They are just lovely kids with excellent manners – which are becoming a rarity these days, but I'm not biased (much)!

I had quite a big sob session at work today; it just gets a bit too much every now and then.

Must go. Lots of love Mum xxxx

***

Christmas day 2000

Dear Kelly,

Well here we are, our first Christmas day without you and it has been absolute hell!

I woke reasonably early this morning and couldn't stay in bed for long, so I got up and continued with the ironing I'd started whilst watching Carols By Candlelight last night. Matt and Quill came and stayed last night, so it was good not to be alone the night before Christmas.

After breakfast this morning, I picked flowers in the misty rain and cried, thinking how awful it was to be picking flowers on Christmas morning for my daughter's grave. Then Dad and I went out to the cemetery and I found it difficult to drive as I was crying so much.

Dad asked me if there was anything wrong and I replied, "Only that my daughter is dead!" He got upset at that, but I felt he should have noticed that I was crying and realised that I was crying for you. However, when we got to the cemetery it was like Bourke Street – there were so many people coming and going – the cemetery is a very popular place on Christmas day.

I left you a bonbon with the flowers, so I hope you were aware that we were thinking of you very much today.

I commented to Fiona earlier that I couldn't believe that you would willingly have put your family through all this pain; I don't believe that you really meant to kill yourself and hurt us all so much. But then again, that is me being selfish I guess.

I am feeling very concerned now, as Fiona went for a walk around the block ages ago and hasn't returned; I hope that nothing has happened to her. That is a new thing with me now, since you went, I don't feel safe – thinking that if you died, then anything can happen to the other children (although they are not children anymore). I worry, worry, worry!

Well I must close and go to bed and sleep (hopefully), I am so very tired and I need to lie down and listen to *My Best Friend's Wedding*, which reminds me so much of you and makes me cry a lot, but that feels good.

I have shed so many tears today, that it seems like I've been crying all day. I love you so much that it just seems wrong that you aren't here.

Catch you later, love Mum xxxx

***

3 January 2001

Dear Kell,

Well here we are at the beginning of another new year, only this one is the first without you. The past few weeks have been very hard, with all the "firsts" and there will be a few more yet to come.

I've wanted to get out to the cemetery for the past few days, but it has been so hot we haven't stirred from the house unless it was absolutely necessary – like going to work.

Work has been interesting, setting up the new clinic in Melbourne, travelling there and still doing my regular work in Geelong when I can. There have been a few upsets at the Melbourne clinic, but they seem to have blown over. Maybe it is just that I'm not coping because of your death. Who knows? Anyway I've done a stack of overtime, which I cannot keep doing.

I haven't been sleeping very well lately, waking really early and unable to go back to sleep. I've been so keyed up, with a feeling of impending doom, a premonition of things to come later in the day perhaps? I hope not really.

So much has been going on, what with Fiona and Damian having difficulties and trying to keep things as normal as possible for Joshua and Hayley. It's a bit like walking a tightrope sometimes. I worry about how Fiona will cope with the kids if she and Damian split up. But I guess I can't do anything about that, just be here for them if they need.

Well it is almost time to go to the gym, my first visit for over two weeks. I've used up all my excuses, so now I'm getting back into it with a vengeance.

Must go now, lots of love Mum xxxx

***

7 January 2001

Dear Kell,

Another milestone gone! Becky's 21st birthday party. It was a great night, they had it at home in the garage. There were tables and umbrellas on the drive, and on the decking they had little tables – the ones Pa made – and chairs. It looked great, especially after dark. There were Christmas lights strung all along the verandah and the house as well as flares in the garden beds along the driveway. The bar was set up in the garage with two girls serving. The food was amazing.

Becky was persuaded to sing some songs for us, which was great. Then everyone was asking for more, so she called for Robyn who came and stood beside me, so I knew then the song would be about you.

Robyn put her arms around me whilst I cried. Mick said she'd written it the week after you died and it was just beautiful, although I didn't really hear all the lyrics as I was crying so much.

All in all it was a great night, but would have been so much better if you'd been there.

Must go now, lots of love Mum xxxx

***

5th February 2001

Dear Kell,

Well it really has been a long time between letters this time. I have not had the strength mentally to write for a while, even though I have given much thought to what I should have been writing at times, there just hasn't been a right time.

Today is a very special day for us – Joshua started school!

It still makes me cry a bit just thinking about it. He was quite excited and very happy to kiss everyone goodbye. Hayley refused to kiss him though – I think she felt that if she did it would be real. She didn't want him to stay there, but she'll be happy when she realises she has got Mummy to herself for the whole day.

He looked great in his new uniform with his huge backpack on – Fiona commented that you could just about fit Hayley in there, but he'll grow into it. It was a happy/sad time seeing him off to school, having been there for his birth and having him stay so much over the last few years; it was almost like sending one of you three kids off to school for the first time.

I missed you so much this week, with all the final preparation for Josh to go to school. You would have loved being there today to see him off too, and I'm sure you would have been there with Fiona when she collects him this afternoon.

Well this is just a short update today, must go now.

Lots of love Mum xxx

***

15 February 2001

Dear Kelly,

Well, once again it has been a long time since I sat to write recent happenings, as well as my feelings on them. This is partly because Dad has been hogging the computer doing his BAS work. He finally finished this quarter today and posted it. It causes a lot of anxiety, plus many hours of extra work – difficult after you've worked a full day on the tools. He is now asleep in the chair in front of the TV.

Things (our relationship) haven't been brilliant between us over the past few weeks; a combination of a lot of things I guess, but we're working on it and I think things will improve now that the BAS is done again.

Fiona and Damian have not been doing so well either, but at last Damian has found somewhere to live and it's just up the road a bit. I think it will be much better for the children and Fiona with the separation. Who knows, they may find they need each other after some time apart. But whatever, they need to separate for a while at least.

It's funny, but they say that many couples break up after a death in the family such as yours, so I guess we are normal after all. Although I'd like to think we will rise above it all eventually.

Dad and I have been together for almost 28 years now it would be a shame if it came to an end. Anyway I'm optimistic that we will get over this hiccup and keep going for the long haul.

Quill is looking very pregnant now, with only just less than eleven weeks to go. I hope she comes a little early so we can all go to Stacey's wedding in May.

We had Murray and Wendy staying here for a couple of days last week on their way to Melbourne. It was lovely seeing them again. Wendy and I took Hayley down to Pako with us and did some shopping – I think Wendy has taught Hayley some bad shopping habits – especially with shoes. Damian took her to get some new shoes and she couldn't decide which ones she wanted – just like Wendy!

Well it's getting too late to keep writing, so I'll close now and maybe write more tomorrow.

Love Mum xxx

***

18 February 2001

Dear Kelly,

Here I am again after just a short break between letters this time. It's either a feast or famine.

I have been doing other writing though. Currently I am attempting to write an account of the day you died and it is very hard to write. I get a few paragraphs written each session until the tears stop me from continuing. I felt I had to start on it before I forget all the little details, although I'm sure I have forgotten many already. However at least I am making the attempt.

Perhaps I'll never actually write that book, but I'd like to think I could give it a damn good try. I think that there is definitely a story there to be told, and that just maybe there are people out there who would like to read it. Maybe I could even help someone by writing it – not the least myself!

I guess deep down I still have a massive inferiority complex that cannot imagine me being clever enough to actually get published. That is there at times for sure; but at other times I feel strong enough and invincible enough to actually write about my experiences. Once I get warmed up with my writing, the words just seem to flow out of me. Will it be like that when I write my book?

Matt came over for a while last night, he seems a bit down again. He and Quill seem to be fighting all the time lately. Shit, what a great legacy you left your family Kell – Fiona and Damian have split up, and not too harmoniously either. Matt and Quill are fighting heaps, which worries me for the baby's sake. Dad and I are having difficulties, which I'm sure will pass. In fact I'm sure all of it will pass soon, just that it is so difficult to accept now.

Gee, Dad and I are only two weeks away from our 28th wedding anniversary, incredible as it seems. Who would have believed we could last this long? It will be a difficult one this time, as it will be the first without you, another in the long list of "firsts" we all have to go through this year, culminating in the first anniversary of your death.

On that note, I think I will stop and get dressed properly for the day.

Lots of love Mum xxx

***

1 April 2001

Dear Kell,

Well it has been a long, long time between drinks! However, it is not as though I haven't been thinking about you. You fill my mind more times that I can tell, and I guess that's the way it will always be now.

Today feels rather special as I am now officially on holidays. Next Saturday Dad and I are flying to Tasmania for a week, which will be great. I have always wanted to visit there. I don't care what the weather is like, just getting away will be great for the both of us, spending some quality time together and relaxing.

Dad has gone out to Marnie and Pa's this morning as there is a guy coming to look at the campervan. Another lady rang from Ballarat yesterday interested in it too. It will be great to sell it, as then we can start paying Marnie and Pa back for your funeral. It is annoying to have that debt hanging over our heads, even though they are not in a hurry for the money, we just want to pay our debts.

The next thing we have to do is select a headstone for your grave. If we sell the camper we will be doing that immediately. Now we just have to decide what to put on the stone.

I would like a photo, and maybe a carving of a fairy. I see you as one now. I like to think you are a fairy visiting little children and looking after them. Probably a silly thought, but that's the way it is. I will always think of you as my little fairy, not destined to stay in this world with us, but to be there in our hearts forever.

Enough of the sentimentality. Yesterday Dad and I went to an Italian wedding – the first we've ever been to. It was the most wonderful day I have had in a long time.

Gosh it feels good to be writing again, I have wanted to do so often, but it hasn't been right to do. I think too that the many long breaks between letters are an indication that I do not need them as much as I did at first. The letters have been a way of coping; I suppose it has almost been denial. If I'm writing to you then you are still around, even though I know you are not here in the flesh, you are in my heart always. So I if I don't write much more to you, then it must mean I am learning to cope without this crutch. It has been my salvation for these last few months, but I think it is time to move on now.

I love you very much. Your loving Mum, forever xxxx

Appendix (ii) Myths About Suicide

MYTH: ***People who talk about killing themselves are not really serious – they are just seeking attention and their behaviour shouldn't be taken seriously***.

REALITY: Anyone who threatens or talks about suicide should always be taken seriously and given support, even if they are not seriously intending to take action at that time.

A person who is distressed enough to discuss suicide or self-harm, needs professional help and support.

MYTH: ***Most suicides occur without warning.***

REALITY: Rarely. Most people thinking about suicide have displayed signs – verbal, nonverbal or even physical. There is often a history of personal problems, mental health issues and even prior attempts.

A person considering suicide may even discuss it with a close friend or family member, some may even seek professional help.

MYTH: ***Girls are not serious about ending their lives when they make suicide attempts***.

REALITY: Girls have higher rates of attempted suicide and boys have higher rates of completed suicide. Girls are not necessarily less serious about their attempts, but may be attracted to less lethal methods. Any suggestion of suicide should be taken seriously.

MYTH: ***People who are suicidal won't ask for help, they just want to be left alone.***

REALITY: Many people who are contemplating suicide will tell someone about their plans.

A significant proportion will visit their doctor in the months prior to an attempt, even though they may not specifically discuss their concerns.

MYTH: ***If someone is determined to end their own life, then there is nothing anyone can do to stop them.***

REALITY: Most people who think about or even attempt suicide can be helped by health professionals, and can be moved to a point where they no longer wish to end their lives. A suicide attempt can often be prevented, by protecting the person at the time and helping them to get professional support.

MYTH: ***People who talk about or attempt suicide are selfish or weak.***

REALITY: People who attempt suicide are usually experiencing strong negative feelings such as depression, fear, anxiety or guilt, and may be suffering from a mental or physical illness. They are often unable to identify any other solution. They need professional help and support, not judgement.

MYTH: ***Talking about suicide with someone you believe may be thinking of it will give them the idea and increase their chances of attempting suicide***.

REALITY: Suicide should not be treated as a taboo subject. Talking about suicide, even asking directly, in a sensitive manner, can give the person the freedom to discuss their distress. Plus it shows that you care. It may also give some relief to them, rather than making them feel worse. It may also prevent suicide and even give the person at risk a greater chance of seeking further help.

MYTH: ***If a person is determined to kill her/himself, then nothing is going to stop them***.

REALITY: Most suicidal people do not want to die. They simply want their pain to go away. Even the most severely depressed person has mixed feelings about dying, and even up to the last moment have mixed thoughts about wanting to die and wanting to live. However overpowering, the impulse to end it all does not last forever.

MYTH: ***If someone tells me they have suicidal thoughts, and asks me not to tell anyone, I am bound by confidentiality***.

REALITY: In the interest of saving life, never promise not to tell anyone. A threat of suicide is one place where confidentiality must be breached. You need to tell others in order to get help, but don't tell anyone who doesn't need to know.

Appendix (iii) Behavioural Warning Signs

These signs are common among people who may be considering suicide:

- Excessive sadness or moodiness: long-lasting sadness, mood swings or unexpected rage.
- Hopelessness: expressing feelings of hopelessness or having little expectation that circumstances can/will improve.
- Withdrawal: spending more time alone; avoiding friends or social activities (possible signs of depression, which is a leading cause of suicide). This includes loss of interest in activities they previously enjoyed.
- Anxiety or agitation: expressions of rage, anger or revenge.
- Expressing feelings of being trapped like there is no way out.
- Sleep problems: not sleeping much or sleeping excessively.
- Dangerous or self-harming behaviour: increased use of drugs and/or alcohol; reckless driving, engaging in unsafe sex. These might indicate that the person no longer values life.
- Making preparations: often when considering suicide as an option, the person will get their affairs in order. This may be in the form of visiting family and friends; giving away personal possessions; making a will; cleaning up room or home; purchasing a firearm;

asking questions such as how do you tie a noose; talking about suicide/death or dying which may also be out of character.

- Changes in personality or appearance: showing a lack of care for appearance – dirty/crushed clothing; hair not washed/brushed; not wearing make-up.

- Sudden calmness: moving from agitation or moodiness/depressive state may be an indication that the decision has been made.

- Threatening suicide: many will give someone a warning sign, but this doesn't necessarily mean they will follow through. Also not everyone who is considering suicide will say so. Every threat of suicide should be taken seriously.

Appendix (iv) Possible Tipping Points

These are where an individual's risk of suicide escalates due to the occurrence of some precipitating event or "tipping point".

Tipping points may be considered the "last straw" that may lead to someone who has previously only been considering suicide, to take action.

Some events or circumstances that may act as tipping points are:

- Recent trauma or life crisis, such as:
  - ~ death of a pet
  - ~ death of a loved one – friend or relative or significant person
  - ~ divorce
  - ~ relationship breakdown
  - ~ diagnosis of a major illness
  - ~ loss of job
  - ~ financial hardship or problems
  - ~ unexpected changes in life circumstances
  - ~ bullying or violence.

Appendix (v) What to Say and What not to Say

When you are concerned that someone may be considering suicide, it is important that you address your concerns. Often it is simply a matter of asking some questions, showing that you care about the person and want to help.

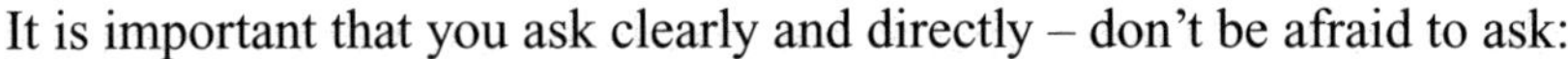

It is important that you ask clearly and directly – don't be afraid to ask:

"Are you thinking about suicide?"

-or-

"Are you thinking of killing yourself?"

-or-

"Sometimes when people are as upset as you seem to be, they may be thinking of suicide. I'm wondering if you're feeling that way?"

-or-

"Sometimes when people have experienced (situation/event) as you have, they have turned to suicide. I'm wondering if you may be feeling that way?"

Whichever question you choose, how you ask the question is less important than that you actually ask the question.

Asking someone if they are thinking of suicide does not increase their risk of suicide.

It is important also to **acknowledge** their feelings, and show that you **care** by asking the question, and then encourage the person to **seek help**.

What not to say

Firstly don't agree to secrecy. It is important that the person gets help, and they may not do it on their own.

- Don't try to cheer them up or jolly them along.
- Don't minimise their feelings; acknowledge their situation.
- Don't moralise, judge or argue with them.
- Don't say that all will be OK.
- Don't try and analyse the "why"; keep their safety in mind.
- Don't argue with them.
- Don't give advice – except to say that help is needed.
- Don't interrupt.
- Don't offer a solution/s.

It is important that you give the person your complete attention, listening intently and showing interest in them.

Be supportive and caring and give them time to speak. If you are not sure of something ask for clarification so you understand what they are saying.

Validate what they are saying.

Perhaps ask what the person has done in the past when they've felt this way, or what could they do to keep themself safe. They may have some ideas themself, but just need encouragement to act on them.

Sources

Hope For Life Suicide Prevention and Bereavement Support

Insight Mental Health Awareness & Suicide Prevention Training

www.suicide.org

www.save.org

www.square.org.au

www.suicideprevention.salvos.org.au

ABOUT THE AUTHOR

Christine Howard

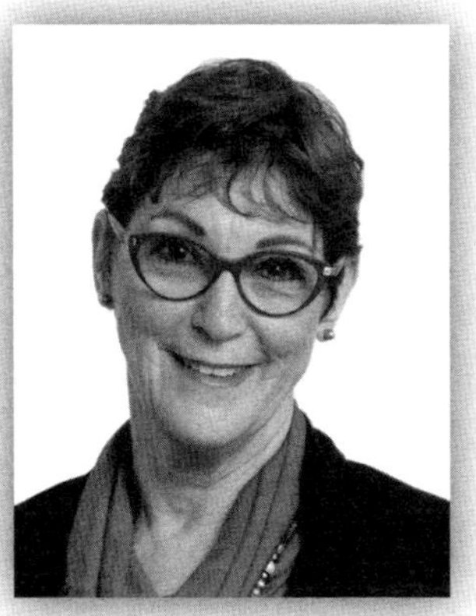

Nurse, massage therapist, entrepreneur, international author

Christine is a nurse, massage therapist, entrepreneur and international author.

Having been born and raised on a remote farm, it wasn't until Christine moved to a small town that she had the opportunity to discover nursing. That was when she spent time working as a cadet nurse in a community hospital.

That experience led her to become a registered nurse after training at Warrnambool Base Hospital. She went on to earn her Diploma of Nursing from the South Australian College of Advanced Education, and her bachelor of Nursing from Flinders University.

Before retiring from a successful nursing career that spanned 32 years, Christine cared for the health of patients at leading hospitals such as Albury Base Hospital, Austin Hospital, Royal Children's Hospital, and St John of God Hospital Geelong.

Throughout her career, Christine continued her health education in a variety of related health fields. She earned a Certificate of Health in

Massage Therapy and a Diploma of Health in Remedial Massage Therapy. She has also completed courses in life coaching and hypnotherapy.

Christine is also an accomplished writer. She was a member of Scribes Writers Geelong and has had her short stories published in *One For'D Road,* a collection of stories which highlighted and celebrated the social life and history of the Ford Motor Company and Geelong people, and *Geelong Rendezvous: An Anthology*.

Now retired from nursing, Christine enjoys spending time writing and managing the family business, Howard Gardening. She launched the garden maintenance and landscaping business in Geelong with her husband and daughter in 1997.

She has travelled throughout China, Hawaii, Kuala Lumpur, Cambodia, New Caledonia and Fiji. While in China, Christine also worked at the Guang An Mien Hospital in Beijing.

Christine Howard is the international author of *Coping With Suicide – Signs We Missed and Strategies to Use in the Aftermath*.

She lives in Geelong, Victoria with her husband Ross.

RECOMMENDED RESOURCES

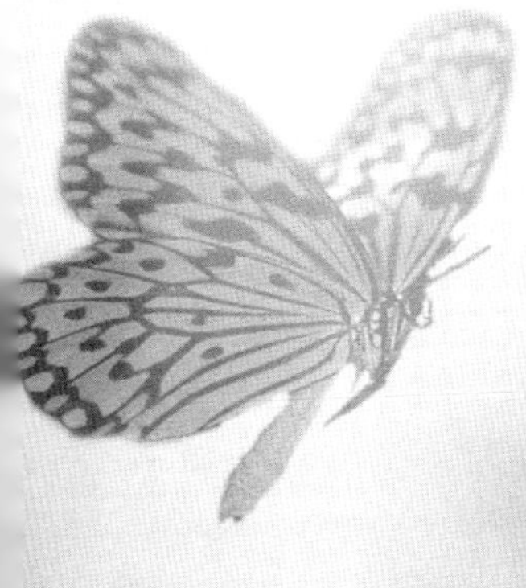

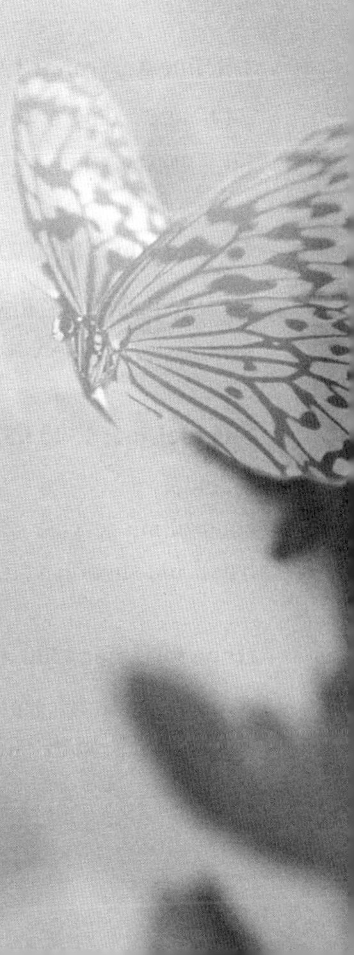

RECOMMENDED RESOURCES

Crisis and Counselling Telephone Lines

Telephone counselling services may be helpful resources for people who have been bereaved by suicide. It can be reassuring to know that there is always a counsellor at the end of the phone to connect with when feelings become overwhelming or you are in need of support. The anonymity and confidentiality of telephone counselling may also appeal to people bereaved by suicide.

Lifeline Australia: 13 11 14

24 hours, 7 days a week

https://www.lifeline.org.au

Beyond Blue: 1300 224 636 24 hours

Call, web chat or email, see www.beyondblue.org.au

Depression, anxiety.

SuicideLine: 1300 651 251

SuicideLine is a 24-hour, Victoria-wide professional telephone counselling service where qualified counsellors are always available to listen and support you.

Hope for Life: 1300 467 354 or 1300 HOPELINE

A nationwide telephone support and referral service specifically for people bereaved by suicide.

Suicide Call Back Service: 1300 659 467

If you find telephone counselling helpful, this may be a suitable service for you. Eligible callers can receive up to six 50-minute counselling sessions with a professional counsellor.

GriefLine: 03 9935 7400

GriefLine is a confidential and free telephone counselling service for anyone experiencing grief.

Veterans Line: 1800 011 046

National helplines and websites

Headspace: 1800 650 890

Free online and telephone service that supports young people aged between 12 and 25 and their families going through a tough time.

Kids Helpline: 1800 55 1800

A free, private and confidential telephone and online counselling service specifically for young people aged between five and 25.

MensLine Australia: 1300 78 99 78

A telephone and online support, information and referral service, helping men to deal with relationship problems in a practical and effective way.

mindhealth*connect*: www.mindhealthconnect.org.au

An innovative website dedicated to providing access to trusted, relevant mental health care services, online programs and resources.

MindSpot Clinic: 1800 61 44 34

An online and telephone clinic providing free assessment and treatment services for Australian adults with anxiety or depression.

Relationships Australia: 1300 364 277

A provider of relationship support services for individuals, families and communities.

SANE Australia Helpline: 1800 18 7263

Information about mental illness, treatments, where to go for support and help for carers.

Suicide and Crisis Support

If you are in an emergency, or at immediate risk of harm to yourself or others, please contact emergency services on 000.

To talk to someone now call:

Lifeline: 13 11 14

Suicide Call Back Service: 1300 659 467

QPR Suicide Prevention Program:

www.suicideprevention.salvos.org.au

QPR is a suicide prevention training program that stands for **"Question, Persuade and Refer".**

Three simple steps that anyone can quickly learn to help save a life from suicide.

People considering suicide often feel very isolated and alone. They may feel that nobody can help them or understand their pain. When unable to see any other way of dealing with pain, suicide may seem to be a way out.

Recognising the warning signs of suicide and learning the skills to help save a life are something that everyone should learn.

Just as people trained in CPR help save thousands of lives each year, people trained in QPR learn how to recognise the warning signs of a suicide crisis and how to question, persuade and refer someone to help.

Reading

Surviving the Hurt by Fiona Lane